The Filaria Sanguinis Hominis and Certain New Forms of Parasitic Disease in India, China, and Warm Countries

PLATE I

Fig. 1

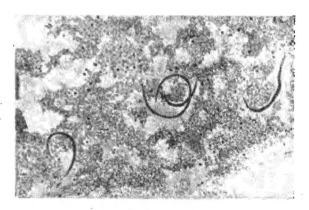

Fig. 2

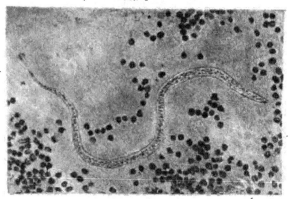

Fig. 3

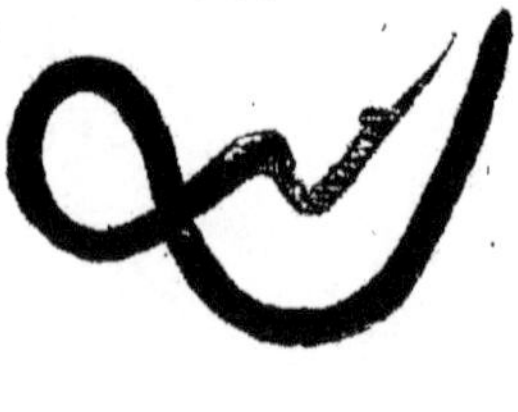

THE

FILARIA SANGUINIS HOMINIS

AND CERTAIN

NEW FORMS OF PARASITIC DISEASE

IN

INDIA, CHINA, AND WARM COUNTRIES

BY

PATRICK MANSON, M.D., C.M.

AMOY, CHINA

LONDON

H. K. LEWIS, 136, GOWER STREET, W.C.

1883

151. 9. 110.

BODLEIAN LIBRARY
4 AUG 83
OXFORD.

PREFACE.

THE subjects treated of in these pages are little understood in Europe. A systematic account of them cannot be found in any text-book or periodical easily accessible to the ordinary medical reader. Nevertheless, they are of great practical and theoretical importance. Any one who takes the trouble to go over the ground is soon convinced of this. I therefore thought that I might do some service to those who desire to work at, or learn about these subjects, and also that I might put others in a favourable position to add to our limited store of knowledge if I brought together into one small volume the gist of certain papers I have published —most of them in the " China Customs Gazette," a practically inaccessible periodical.

Chapter I. is a reprint of a paper contributed to the "Pathological Society's Transactions" for 1881 (vol. xxxii.). In it, as a sort of comment on a lymph-scrotum exhibited to the Society, I have given a *précis* of our knowledge of the life-history of *filaria sanguinis hominis*, and of its pathological significance. In the succeeding five chapters, and in foot-notes,

I have given a more detailed account of the evidence
on which I found my conclusions. I have been
careful to do this as many, who have not taken the
trouble to work out the subject in detail for themselves, have questioned my facts, and, of course,
denied my conclusions.   The life-history of this
parasite is so complicated, and its demonstration involves so much patient labour, that one must not
be unprepared for this : a long time may elapse
before accumulated confirmations have brought about
the general acceptance of the facts I have described.
Sceptics who have the opportunity of working ought
to work and collect evidence before they contradict
or offer anything but a very qualified opinion.

Endemic hæmoptysis and tinea imbricata are
both new and interesting diseases.

The short note on the parasite called after me
by my friend Dr. Cobbold, I have introduced in the
hope that those who have the chance of post-mortem
examinations in Orientals may look for the animal.
What pathological importance it may possess I cannot
say; probably it will turn out to be only a helminthological curiosity.

The parasitic diseases, apart from any special
interest attaching to them, possess many instructive
and suggestive analogies to the more widely-spread
and deadly zymotic diseases. Such facts as filarial
periodicity, the action of intermediary hosts in the
spread of communicable but non-infectious disease, the
embolism of the lymph-channels by the aborted ova
of the filaria—the disease of a disease, so to speak—

ought to be full of significance to the general pathologist. Analogies to the ordinary zymotic diseases
cannot fail to occur to the attentive student of the
parasitic diseases, and I trust these pages will
supply one or two facts which may aid in throwing light on some obscure problems in pathology.

From the knowledge we now possess of the life-
history of their exciting causes, it is quite possible
to prevent, and, in time, to stamp out the elephantoid diseases and endemic hæmoptysis. Undoubtedly, did these diseases affect European
countries, by this time practical sanitarians would
have been at work. Unfortunately they affect the
natives of countries in which we have but a very
secondary interest, and who are themselves absolutely indifferent to sanitary matters. But one can
understand how, by hindering the access of the
mosquito to drinking-water, or by filtration, or
cooking, we might prevent the elephantoid diseases,
and how by similar means we might put an end
to endemic hæmoptysis. In the life-history of
most of the parasites of which we possess a little
knowledge, there is a weak point where man may
step in and arrest development. May we not hope
from this, that when we know more of the life of
other and more deadly disease-germs, a weak point
in their histories also may be found inviting the
attack of the sanitarian?

My readers will not fail to be struck with the
crudeness and incomplete character of much of my
work. In deprecation of their criticism I would

ask them to remember that I worked under many disadvantages. Besides the constant interruptions incident to private practice, I had to contend with disadvantages unknown to my more fortunate co-labourers at home. The absence of a good library, of competent assistants, of friendly advice and criticism, are serious obstacles to successful work; added to these, the depressing influence of a hot climate, and the prejudices of my native patients, had to be fought against. I trust, therefore, in criticising my work some allowance will be made for these circumstances.

I take this opportunity to thank Sir Joseph Fayrer, F.R.S., and Dr. Spencer Cobbold, F.R.S., for many acts of kindness. To them I am much indebted for bringing my work before the profession in England, and by the stamp of their approval gaining for it a hearing. I have also to thank Dr. Stephen Mackenzie for the use of the beautiful micro-photographs of the filaria forming the frontispiece, and for his successful efforts in confirming the discovery of filarial periodicity.

P. M.

Amoy, China,
    June, 1883.

CONTENTS.

CHAPTER VI.

CHAPTER VII.

CHAPTER VIII.

CHAPTER IX.

ILLUSTRATIONS.

PLATE I (Frontispiece).

Fig. 1.—Four filariæ, as seen in the blood, at an enlargement of about 70 diameters.

Fig. 2.—A filaria at an enlargement of about 270 diameters. The granular appearance of the body is a post-mortem change.

Fig. 3.—Filaria at an enlargement of about 270 diameters, stained with anilin, showing partial retraction from external sheath.

PLATE II.

METAMORPHOSIS OF THE FILARIA IN THE MOSQUITO.

When the number of hours is alluded to, it is meant to express only the number of hours from the time the mosquito was captured to the time its abdomen was opened. As it would be impossible to say when a given mosquito fed, whether early in the evening, at midnight, or towards morning, a latitude of from one to nine hours must be granted in estimating the time the filaria has been subjected to the influence of its intermediary host.

Fig. 1.—The filaria a short time after ingestion by the mosquito. Movements vigorous, but slowing down. Lash, and oral movements distinct.

Fig. 2.—Movements very languid; sheath separated by an appreciable interval from the body, which is transversely striated: from three to six hours after ingestion.

Fig. 3.—Eight hours: Movements still more languid; the sheath has disappeared; transverse striation and oral pouting very distinct. I note of a specimen examined about twenty-six hours after ingestion: "Many specimens dead; one more active than the others showed oral movements; the transverse striation distinct, and inside this many dark and shining specks seen moving as if in a fluid."

ILLUSTRATIONS.

PLATE II.—*Continued.*

FIG. 4.—Dead and probably undergoing degeneration or digestion.

FIG. 5.—Thirty-six hours after capture of mosquito: Movement intermitting, but distinct and often vigorous; faint indication
of a double outline; body granular; jointed nature of
caudal appendage very evident.

FIG. 6.—Thirty-six hours after capture: Tail distinctly differentiated;
breadth of body $\frac{1}{2000}$-in. Specimens very similar to this
were found up to sixty hours, with tail rather more distinctly differentiated, a faint double outline, and an obscure
convoluted-like arrangement in the interior of the body.

FIG. 7.—Thirty-nine hours: Length, $\frac{1}{90}$-in.; breadth, $\frac{1}{2500}$-in. No
mouth or striation visible; faint double outline; hardly any
granules in interior, except about the head, where they
are faint and fine; intermitting but vigorous flexion of
the tail, and perhaps slight movement of body.

FIG. 8.—Forty-nine hours: Specimens like this embedded in oily, white,
digested-looking material. Still blood in mosquito's
stomach, but the embryos in this all dead. In the specimen represented the body is thick and finely granular;
the granules are shining, and have a faint though quite
distinct movement.

FIG. 9.—Fifty hours: Faint caudal movements; no striation, granula-
tion, or structure of any sort visible.

FIG. 10.—Sixty-three hours: Body homogeneous; slight indication only
of a tail; thicker and shorter; one specimen shows faint
indication of striation. To one slide water was added, and
pretty vigorous movement followed, and the tail was again
seen.

PLATE III.

METAMORPHOSIS OF THE FILARIA IN THE MOSQUITO—*Continued.*

FIG. 1.—Seventy to ninety hours (4th day): Many specimens like that
represented; tail particularly distinct, some indication of a
mouth with lips; some specimens are quite structureless
in the interior, whereas in others an indistinct convoluted
appearance can be made out; all are quite motionless.

FIG. 2.—5th day: Nearly all mosquitos are dead, their ova having
been deposited on the water. In a living mosquito embryos
as at Fig. 1; in another mosquito many embryos as at
Fig. 2; a distinct four-lipped mouth visible; with a high
power a double outline is easily made out, and it becomes
apparent that the tail is merely an integumental appendage.
Indications of alimentary canal.

ILLUSTRATIONS.

PLATE III.—*Continued.*

FIG. 3.—5th day : Body elongating; granular or cell-like appearance in interior; indications of an anus.

FIG. 4.—5th and 6th day : Body still longer; posterior end swelling; granular matter escaping from anus; alimentary canal distinctly indicated; tail shrinking, but still occasionally exhibiting movements of flexion and extension.

FIG. 5.—From mosquito on the 6th day : Body of developing embryo short and stumpy; mouth, alimentary canal, and anus distinct; in two the tail has disappeared; in one some slight indications of it remain; bodies filled with large cells; larger cells posteriorly.

FIG. 6.—5th to 6th day: Body broader and more elongated; tail, a mere stump; mouth, alimentary tube, œsophagus, valve, and intestine very distinct; head and fore-part of the body rocked backwards and forwards in rapid swaying motion.

FIG. 7.—5th to 6th day: Body now the thirtieth of an inch in length, very transparent; the animal in constant motion, rushing backwards and forwards through the water, and forcing obstacles of all sort aside. Drawn on a smaller scale.

FIG. 8.—Head and tail of No. 7, the animal being restrained and crushed by pressure on the cover glass. (*a*) The head is seen to be crowned with four strong circumoral papillæ (the boring apparatus); the ruptured end of the œsophagus protrudes where the body has been torn across, and in front of this a faint line is seen emerging on the surface of the integument, and is probably the rudiment of uterus and vagina. (*b*) The alimentary canal is seen to enter the ruptured end of the tail. No anus visible. Caudal appendage completely disappeared.

PLATE IV.

Lymph-scrotum and elephantiasis scroti; lymphatic glands of the groin and lymphatics of scrotum varicose.—Case VII.

PLATE V.

Elephantiasis of leg and operation flaps supervening in a case in which a lymph-scrotum had been excised.—Case XVIII.

PLATE VI.

Elephantiasis of the leg, varicose groin-glands, and lymph-scrotum combined.—Case XIX.

ILLUSTRATIONS.

PLATE VII.

Elephantiasis of the leg; lymphous discharge from calf of leg: varicose groin-glands; chyluria.—Case XXI.

PLATE VIII.

OVA OF DISTOMA RINGERI, AND DEVELOPMENT OF THE EMBRYO.

FIGS. 1, 2, 3.—Ova newly expectorated.

FIGS. 4, 5, 6, 7, 8, 9.

PLATE IX.

OVA OF DISTOMA RINGERI, AND DEVELOPMENT OF THE EMBRYO— *Continued.*

FIGS. 1 and 2.—Ova after washing and immersion in fresh water for various periods; segmentation and gradual development of embryo.

FIG. 3.—Embryo in ovum soon after appearance of cilia; movement commencing.

FIG. 4.—The same after extrusion from ovum by pressure; the beak protruding; large globules appearing in the body; death approaching.

FIG. 5.—The shell from which an embryo has escaped; the operculum thrown back.

FIGS. 6, 7, 8, 9.—The free embryo, assuming various shapes according to the character of movement it is indulging in.

PLATE X.

THE FUNGUS OF TINEA IMBRICATA.

FIGS. 1 to 7.—Drawn from specimens treated with liquor potassæ and stained with vesuvin brown.

FIG. 8.—Stained with saffranin.

WOODCUTS.

PAGE 25.—Woodcut showing the stretching of its chorional envelope by the embryo of the *filaria corvi torquati.*

PAGE 128.—Fragment of female *filaria sanguinis hominis* from abscess in thigh.

[illegible]

[illegible]

[illegible]

PLATE [illegible]

[illegible] dark [illegible]

[illegible]

PLATE [illegible]

[illegible] stomach [illegible]

[illegible]

[illegible] accordance [illegible]

[illegible] the [illegible]

[illegible] which [illegible] the operculum [illegible]

[illegible] movement [illegible]

PLATE X.

[illegible]

[illegible] liquor potassæ [illegible]

[illegible]

[illegible]

[illegible] torquata.

[illegible] from disease.

PLATE II.

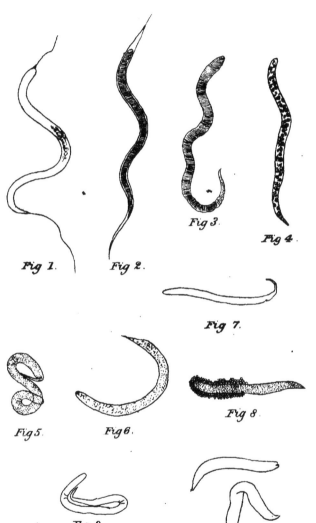

Fig 1.

Fig 2.

Fig 3.

Fig 4.

Fig 7.

Fig 5.

Fig 6.

Fig 8.

Fig 9.

Fig 10.

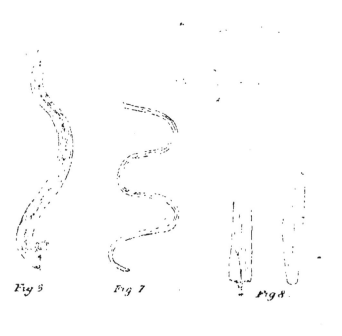

Fig 5   Fig 7   Fig 8.

PLATE III.

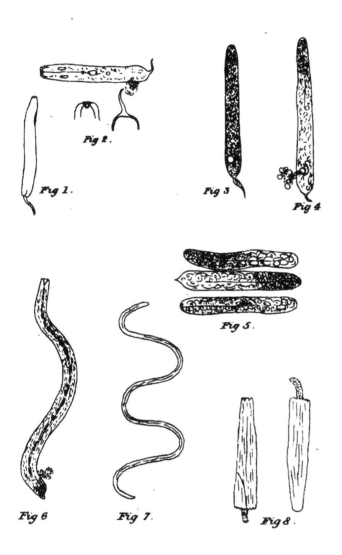

Fig 1.

Fig 2.

Fig 3

Fig 4

Fig 5.

Fig 6

Fig 7.

Fig 8

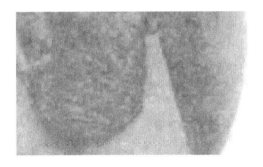

PLATE IV

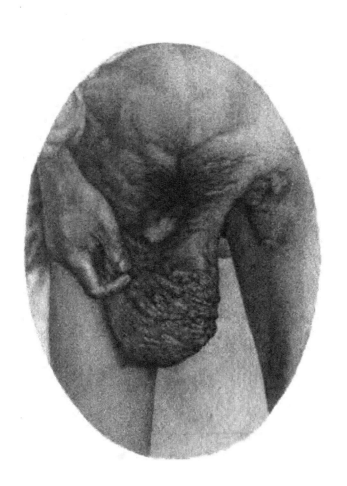

Fig. 3

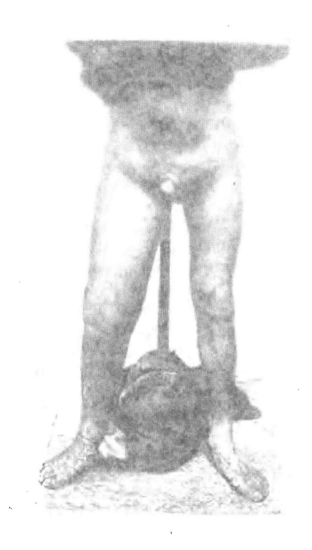

PLATE V.

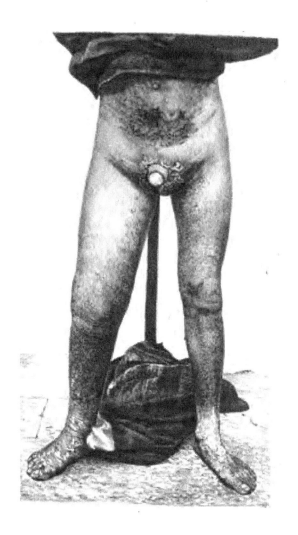

PLATE VI.

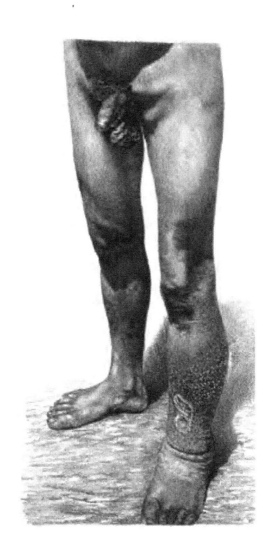

PLATE VI.

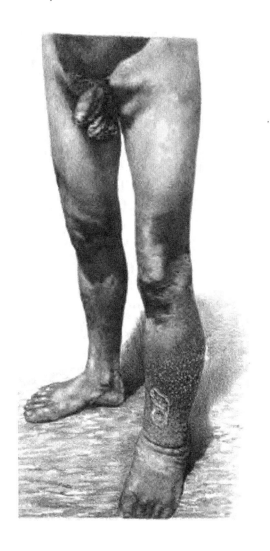

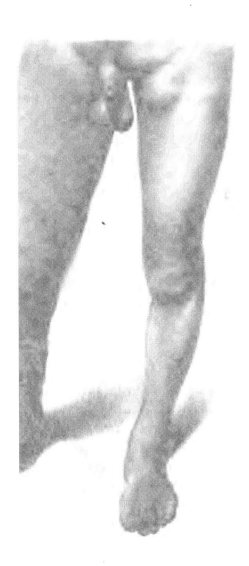

PLATE VII

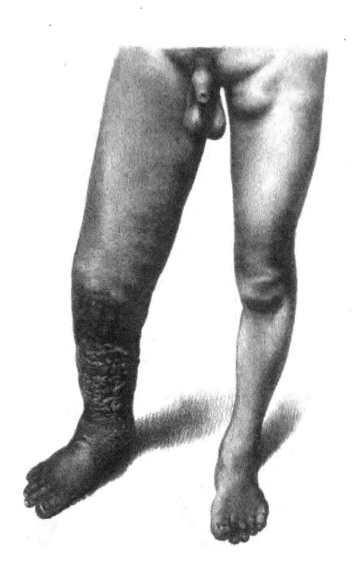

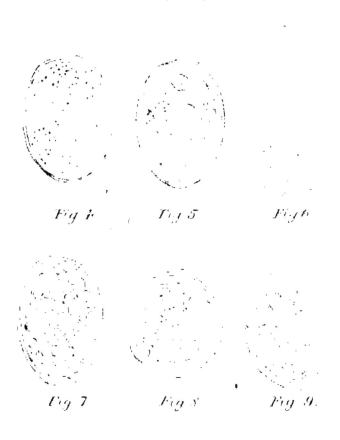

Fig 4.   Fig 5   Fig 6

Fig 7   Fig 8   Fig 9.

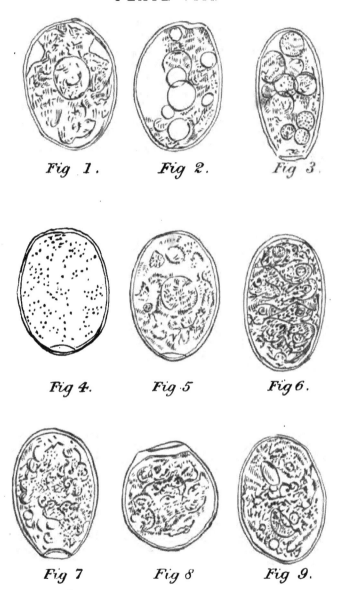

PLATE VIII.

Fig 1.   Fig 2.   Fig 3.

Fig 4.   Fig 5   Fig 6.

Fig 7   Fig 8   Fig 9.

Fig. 7. 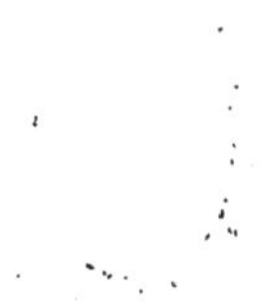　　　　　*Fig.* 8.　　　　*Fig.* 9

PLATE IX.

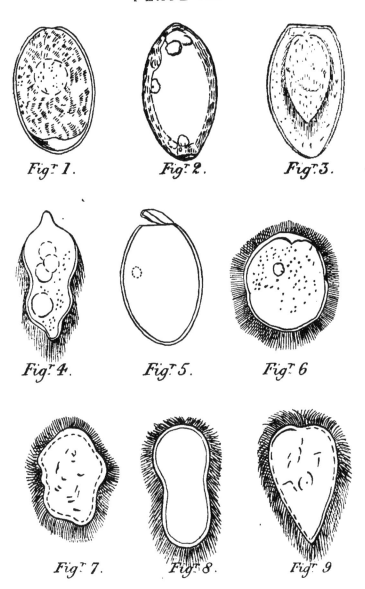

Fig.ᵀ 1.   Fig.ᵀ 2.   Fig.ᵀ 3.

Fig.ᵀ 4.   Fig.ᵀ 5.   Fig.ᵀ 6

Fig.ᵀ 7.   Fig.ᵀ 8.   Fig.ᵀ 9

Fig 7 × 530

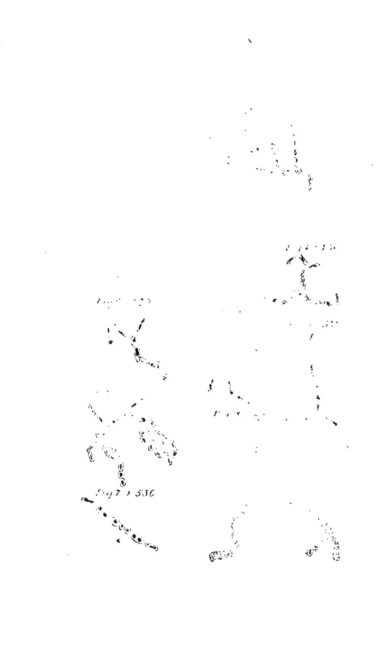

PLATE X.

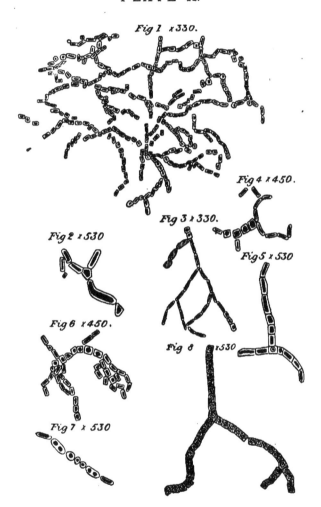

Fig 1 x330.

Fig 4 x450.

Fig 3 x330.

Fig 2 x530

Fig 5 x530

Fig 6 x450.

Fig 8   x530

Fig 7 x 530

THE

FILARIA SANGUINIS HOMINIS.

CHAPTER I.

THE FILARIA SANGUINIS HOMINIS, AND ITS
PATHOLOGICAL SIGNIFICANCE.[*]

THE preparation exhibited to the Society on May
17th, by Dr. Thin, as an example of the disease I
have called lymph-scrotum,[†] is unique. For although
lymph-scrotum is common enough in certain countries, and as a morbid preparation has occasionally
been exhibited in Europe, and the parent of the
hæmatozoon, named by Lewis *filaria sanguinis
hominis*, has been found by at least four observers,
yet I believe this is the first instance in which
the parasite has been found in its proper habitat,
a lymphatic vessel, and has been seen *in situ*.[‡]

[*] This chapter is a reprint of a paper contributed to the
"Pathological Society's Transactions" for 1881, vol. xxxii.

[†] This disease has received various names, as varix
lymphaticus, nævoid elephantiasis, etc. Lymph-scrotum is
shorter and more expressive.

[‡] For a full report of this case, see p. 123.

The man from whom this lymph-scrotum was removed last October, had suffered from symptoms of lymphatic obstruction for about five years. At intervals lymph was discharged from vesicles on the surface of the scrotum, and for the last three years the discharge had been almost constant. The usual and characteristic vesicles covered the lower part of the scrotum, the tissues of which were thickened, but not indurated or greatly enlarged; to the touch they felt soft and spongy. The groin glands on both sides were enlarged, and felt indurated, or rather as if an indurated nucleus was surrounded by a spongy and varicose cortex. The clear and straw-coloured coagulable lymph contained embryo filariæ; but, though frequently searched, blood from the finger contained no parasites. The man's spleen was considerably enlarged, and he was intensely anæmic. As there seemed no prospect of the lymphorrhagia ceasing, to save his life I was compelled to remove the scrotum. Before operating I ventured to prognosticate that the parent filaria would be found in the part removed. That I was justified in making this prognostication was proved by the parasite appearing on the cut surfaces of the scrotum in active movement. It turned out to be a female. Half of the animal lay in a dilated lymphatic, and is still there; for, on attempting to withdraw it, the body snapped across. Probably the male is there also.

In order to make clear the reasons for the prognostication I made, it is necessary to examine the entire subject of *filaria sanguinis hominis*, and its connection with certain diseases—a subject as yet little understood, but one destined, both from its scientific interest and vast practical importance, to occupy no insignificant place in pathology.

Its enormous practical importance will be comprehended when I state that wherever elephantiasis * is endemic this parasite is to be found; that elephantiasis is endemic over half the globe, at least over that part of the globe where the major part of mankind resides; that this parasite produces a group of diseases, very common in these countries, which, though not commonly fatal, do sometimes kill, and always give rise to much pain, deformity, and inconvenience; that it is in our power completely to prevent the access of the animal to the tissues of man, and thereby prevent these diseases; and that this desirable result can be attained by the simplest of means. These seem sweeping statements, but the sequel, I am convinced, will fully bear me out in making them.

For a complete account of the gradual progress of our knowledge of this parasite I would refer the reader to Cobbold's recently-published work on "Parasites."† There the history of the subject is given, along with an exhaustive bibliography, down to the date of the publication of his work. I will confine myself to stating only so much of the history as is necessary to understanding the subject, and will avoid, as much as possible, everything that appears to me unimportant or doubtful.

* When the term elephantiasis is used, elephantiasis arabum is meant; never elephantiasis græcorum or leprosy.

† "Parasites: a Treatise on the Entozoa of Man and Animals." By T. Spencer Cobbold, M.D., F.R.S. London, 1879.

The animal I saw wriggling on the cut surface of the scrotum shown to the society, and half of whose body is still lying in the lymphatic vessel it occupied during life, is the parent of an embryo nematode, first found in chylous urine by Wucherer in 1866, and in the blood by Lewis in 1872, and named by the latter observer *filaria sanguinis hominis*. The embryo was discovered several years before the mature animal, for it was not till 1876 that Bancroft in Australia, and a few months later, in 1877, Lewis in India, found the parent worm. Since then the mature animal has been found by Araujo and dos Santos in Brazil, and by myself in China, and has been named by Cobbold *Filaria Bancrofti*. Only a small part of the male worm has hitherto been found, and as in this case it was intimately associated with the female, it is extremely probable that the sexes live together. Like the males of most filariæ it was considerably smaller than the female. The latter is a long, slender, hair-like animal, quite three inches in length, but only $\frac{1}{100}$-in. in breadth, of an opaline appearance, looking as it lies in the tissues like a delicate thread of catgut animated and wriggling. A narrow alimentary canal runs from the simple club-like head to within a short distance of the tail, the remainder of the body being almost entirely occupied by reproductive organs. The vagina opens about $\frac{1}{25}$-in. from the head; it is very short, and bifurcates into two uterine horns, which, stuffed with embryos at all stages of development, run backwards nearly to the tail. Under the microscope fully-formed embryos, just as we see them in the blood, can be seen escaping from the vagina. The animal is therefore viviparous.

For further details on the structure of the parent worm Lewis's and Cobbold's writings should be consulted.* Here I may not occupy space with helminthological detail unnecessary for the full understanding of my argument; but there is one point it would be well to settle before proceeding with the history of the parasite, and that is, the exact position occupied by the mature animal in the human body— what tissue or vessel.

The preparation shown to the Society is almost sufficient to settle this. In it, when fresh, and immediately after its removal from the body, the animal was seen protruding from the cut end of a lymphatic vessel from which it had partly crept out; the other end of the dilated vessel was seen in the face of the wound, and from it, the groin-glands being pressed with the hand, lymph was seen to regurgitate. Even prior to this the lymphatics were credited with being the proper habitat of the animal, for in many cases of lymph-scrotum, chyluria, and varicose groin-glands, its young have been found in the lymph.† It might have been objected to this, as a conclusive argument, that possibly those embryos found their way into the lymphatics by escaping from the capillaries. This is extremely unlikely; yet, admitting its possibility in the case of the free embryo, such a feat would be impossible to the ovum both on account

---

* "The Microscopic Organisms found in the Blood of Man and Animals, and their Relation to Disease." By Timothy Richard Lewis, M.B. Reprinted from the "Fourteenth Annual Report of the Sanitary Commissioner with the Government of India," 1877.

† See many of the cases related in chapters iv. and v.

of its diameter and its being a perfectly passive body. Ova, however, have been found in the lymph,* and the ovum being too large to pass from the outside to the inside of a lymphatic, and having no power to work its way, the parent that laid it must have communicated directly with the lymphatics. Again, in not a few instances filaria embryos have been found in the lymph discharges of individuals from whose blood not a single specimen could be obtained;† they could not, therefore, have come from the blood-vessels. It may be taken as settled that the parent worm lives in the lymphatics.

Thus, then, the parent filaria lying in a lymphatic vessel emits her young into the lymph-stream; along this they are carried to the lymphatic glands. As they are only about $\frac{1}{3000}$-in. in diameter, no broader than many of the lymph-corpuscles that accompany them, they have no difficulty in entering and traversing the minute vessels into which the afferent lymphatic divides. For the same reason, and by virtue of its vigorous movements, it passes the parenchyma of the gland, and emerging into the efferent vessels is borne along the current till, having traversed gland after gland, it finds itself in the thoracic duct, and finally in the blood itself.

As found there, and also in the lymph, this nematode embryo when examined by a high microscopic power is seen to be a long, slender, snake-like, gracefully-shaped animal, possessed of an activity so great that until paralysed by approaching

* See Case XXIV. p. 130; and Case XXV. p. 131.
† See Case XIV. p. 103; Case XX. p. 115; Case XXI. p. 116; Case XXII. p. 123.

death or inspissation of the medium it lies in measurements and observations of structure can hardly be made. It measures about $\frac{1}{90}$-in. $\times \frac{1}{3500}$-in., is perfectly transparent, and apparently structureless. The anterior part of the body tapers slightly, and at its very extremity a pouting movement, as if of breathing, is to be detected. Posteriorly the body gradually tapers down to a fine point, the extreme end of which in most specimens has the look of being articulated, for this part does not always harmonize with the general curve of the body, but seems bent at an angle. In some individuals a brown aggregation of granular matter can be detected about the centre of the body half way between head and tail. An extremely delicate sac encloses the animal, fitting it accurately; but as this sac is about one-third longer than the body it is unoccupied and collapsed into the semblance of a lash at the head, or tail, or both, according to the position or direction of movement of its contents. If the animal is rushing forward, the anterior part of the sac is occupied and a long lash of collapsed sac dangles from the tail; if the animal is retreating tail first, then this part of the sac is occupied and the superfluous integument trails after the head. (Plate I.)

If a man in whose blood this parasite has been found is kept constantly under observation for a number of days, and freshly-drawn specimens of his blood examined at short intervals, it will soon be evident that the parasite is not equally abundant at all times; in fact, that often it is entirely absent. Sometimes slide after slide will be examined without a single specimen being discovered, notwithstanding that a few hours before the parasite could be found by the hundred in every drop of blood. If a register of these observations is kept it will presently be apparent that there is a diurnal periodicity in this presence and absence of embryos in the general circulation. It will be found that during the day, unless under peculiar circumstances, they are entirely absent; that about six or seven o'clock in the evening, with "military-like punctuality," as Cobbold expresses it, they march to their night quarters; gradually, as night advances their numbers increase; by twelve o'clock as many as 100, or even more, may be counted in every drop of blood. About this time their numbers reach their maximum, and then, as morning approaches, they become fewer and fewer; by eight or nine a.m. they entirely disappear. From nine a.m. to six p.m. very rarely is it possible to procure a single specimen. The only thing that interrupts the regularity of this periodicity is an attack of fever. If this does not occur it is maintained day after day. I have watched it preserve its rhythm for a month on end, and there is no reason for supposing that, but for the exception mentioned, it is ever interrupted.* This is a most remarkable phenomenon, and one as yet unaccounted for. But though we may not be able to explain it we understand its object, for night is the time when at the surface of the body the embryo has an opportunity of advancing in its development.†

* This was written before Dr. Stephen Mackenzie showed that periodicity was affected by altering the hours for sleeping.

† For a full account of filarial periodicity the reader is referred to chap. ii., and to Dr. Stephen Mackenzie's paper on

There appears to be no reason for supposing that after the embryo leaves the uterus of its parent, and as long as it remains in the body of the original host, there is any advance in development. As seen in the blood all look much alike; and, indeed, it is evident that any degree of growth would be incompatible with the life of the human host. Such a swarm of animalcules did they but each attain a hundredth part of the size of their parents would soon make life impossible. For this reason, as well as for the reason that the species to be continued must pass into other men, the embryo must leave the original host. But how? Only on rare occasions have they been found in the excretions, and then only in those of a morbid character.

Nature is not likely to trust to the accident of a disease for the continuation of a species. Her operations are always orderly and reveal a plan. She may be careless of the single life, but she is very careful of the species. Seeing, then, that there is no provision made in the structure of the embryo for its spontaneously escaping from the body, and that this escape must be effected, it follows that some outside influence must bring this about.

In the somewhat analogous parasite, *trichina spiralis*, such an opportunity is afforded by the animal that devours the flesh of the original host.

" A Case of Filarial Hæmato-chyluria," in the " Transactions of the Pathological Society of London," 1882, vol. xxxiii.; also to a very interesting paper on " Filaria Disease in South Formosa," by Dr. W. Wykeham Myers, in the " China Customs Medical Reports," for the half-year ended March 31st, 1881; 21st issue.

But in few countries is human flesh consumed in so wholesale a fashion as would warrant us supposing the *filaria sanguinis hominis* was similarly treated.

As the embryo parasite lives in the blood it is likely that the first step in its development and towards freedom will be given it by something that abstracts the blood. Thus, then, the privilege will be confined to a very limited number of animals— the blood-suckers. This includes the fleas, lice, bugs, leeches, mosquitos, and sand - flies. But as the parasite is confined to a limited area of the earth's surface it is more than likely that this friend of the filaria has a corresponding and limited distribution. Fleas, lice, bugs, leeches, as they are found pretty well all the world over, must therefore be excluded.

Reasoning in this way I concluded in the summer of 1877 * that either the mosquito or the sand-fly liberated the parasite. Had I been aware then of the nocturnal habits of the worm I would have excluded the sand-fly likewise. In this way, then, reasoning from its faculty of piercing the blood-vessels, its nocturnal habits, and its geographical distribution, the mosquito appears of all animals the most suited to assist the parasite. And as there are many species of mosquitos everywhere in the tropics, and in many other parts of the world, but filaria disease is limited, it follows that every species of mosquito will not answer; it must be a species similarly limited. I know of several tropical species that are impotent to assist the parasite; but there is at least one species

* "China Customs Medical Reports," No. 14, 1878; "Linnæan Society's Journal of Zoology," vol. xiv. p. 304.

possessing all the necessary qualifications, and which others, as well as myself, have over and over again proved to be an efficient intermediary host for *filaria sanguinis hominis*.* The female of this particular species of culex (it is with her alone we have to deal, the male, owing to the construction of his oral appendages, being incapable of piercing the skin) is a small, dark-brown insect, about $\frac{3}{8}$-in. in length. She may be recognized by her size, her colour, and the entire absence of pronounced markings on her abdomen, thorax, or legs. Her head is small and dark, and carries a proboscis about two-thirds the length of her body, dark, too, like the head, strong, and slightly bulbous at the free extremity. About sunset the sexes leave their retreat, and for an hour or two wheel about in the air, generally, when in a house, near the ceiling. About eight o'clock they descend in search of food, and the female greedily avails herself of the blood of the first animal in which she can fix her proboscis, be it man or beast. About two minutes suffice, if she is not disturbed, to fill the stomach. She then retires to some shady place, if possible in the vicinity of water, and during four or five days is occupied in digesting her single meal and maturing her ova. When this is

* Lewis: op. cit. ; Araujo (see Cobbold's " Parasites," p. 198) ; Bancroft (" Diseases of Plants and Animals," etc. ; a pamphlet published in Brisbane, Australia). Dr. Sonsino, of Cairo, Egypt, wrote me lately saying that he also had recently observed the metamorphosis of the filaria in the mosquito. Specimens of filaria-impregnated mosquitos I sent home some years ago to Dr. Cobbold, have on several occasions been exhibited at different medical and scientific societies in London.

completed she betakes herself to the water, and on
the surface of this deposits two little boat-shaped
masses of eggs.   After effecting this she dies.

If, then, a female of this particular species of
mosquito pierces the skin of a filaria-infested subject,
the proboscis, buried in the blood-stream, is speedily
beset by the embryos.   These as they are carried
along by the current become entangled by their
lashes,* and are then transferred in great abundance,

---

* Many of the hæmatozoa of the lower animals which I have
studied are, unlike that of man, quite naked and unprovided
with a sheath or lash.   This arrangement probably has
reference to the well-being of the parasite.   The purpose of
the lash in *filaria sanguinis hominis* is, doubtless, to assist in its
transferrence to the stomach of the mosquito in the way I
describe.   Occasionally I have had an opportunity of making
an experiment which goes a long way to prove this.   A not
infrequent accompaniment of filaria disease, perhaps the only
symptom of it, is that sort of dropsy of the tunica vaginalis
which has been called "galactocele"; properly it should be called
"lymphocele."   In this affection the congested lymphatics
relieve themselves by rupture into the tunica vaginalis, and
we have accordingly a collection of filaria-bearing lymph in
this sac.   Such a condition may be suspected when the glands
of the groin are much enlarged and varicose, and the swelling of the testicle does not transmit light as in ordinary
hydrocele.   If now we tap such a "lymphocele," instead of
the clear fluid of a hydrocele we get milky lymph such as
escapes from ordinary lymph-scrotum, and in the sediment of
this lymph filaria embryos are to be found in great abundance.
As a rule, the lymph after withdrawal coagulates very
rapidly, but in a certain proportion of cases coagulation does
not occur.   I do not know the reason for this absence of the
coagulating property.   I have met with such cases more than
once.   If a sample of this non-coagulating filariated lymph
is procured, and into it is dropped a few fibres of cotton wool,

along with the blood, to the stomach of the insect.
Here for a time they continue their movements;
but gradually, as the blood coagulates and becomes
digested, motion is restricted, and finally, but for an
intermitting jerk of the tail, entirely ceases. Some
are digested or expelled in the fæces. A favoured
few, however, survive, and enter on a very interesting metamorphosis. First, the hitherto smooth and
perfectly structureless body becomes marked by
delicate and closely-set transverse striæ, as if from
general longitudinal shrinking; and the bag in which it
has hitherto been tightly enveloped appears separated
from it by an appreciable interval, and possibly finally
disappears. Then the striæ lose their distinctness,
and the body of the animal seems as if it became
broader, shorter, and filled with a fluid containing
granular matter and exhibiting to-and-fro movements. The extreme tip of the tail, probably that
portion of it described as if articulated to the rest

it will be found that after a few minutes the cotton will sink
to the bottom of the vessel containing the lymph. It should
be allowed to remain there for some time, and then fished out
with a needle and transferred to the stage of the microscope.
If the experiment has been successful, it will be found that
hundreds and thousands of filariæ now beset the fibres of the
cotton wound about it in every possible fashion, in groups, in
lines, and singly, most of them being attached by their head
or tail lashes which are wound firmly round the fibres.
Where a kink or knot occurs, or where two or three fibres
cross or interlace, there is sure to be a thick cluster of filariæ;
reminding one by its appearance and the wriggling, snake-
like movements of the parasites, of the head of the Gorgon.
Doubtless the little worms become attached to the proboscis
of the mosquito as they do to the cotton fibres in the experiment.

of the body, does not partake in the general broad-
ening, but looks like an appendage stuck on to the
sausage-shaped mass; at short intervals it exhibits
sudden and vigorous movements of flexion and
extension. By-and-by minute cell-like bodies appear
and arrange themselves along a line now beginning
to be visible in the centre of the cylinder, and
opening near, but a little in advance of the tail at
one end, and at the semblance of a mouth at the
other. At this stage the animal is perfectly passive,
and its caudal appendage shortens and disappears.
Growth now commences, and with growth a swaying
movement of the anterior part of the body. As
growth progresses movement increases, and finally,
when the little animal has attained a length of about
$\frac{1}{50}$-in., it exhibits prodigious activity, rushing forwards and backwards indifferently, and thrusting
every obstacle aside. If by pressure we restrain its
movements, or fracture its delicate body, its head
is seen to be crowned with three or four nipple-like
papillæ; an alimentary canal is visible running from
mouth to anus, and rudiments of generative organs
can likewise be traced.* (Plates II and III.)

* It may be useful to those who wish to repeat and test my
observations to know the plan I found most successful in procuring filaria-bearing mosquitos, and how their bodies were
afterwards treated for microscopic examination. One must be
careful to procure the proper species of mosquito, and be
assured that it has fed on filariated *human* blood. If any
mosquito is caught at random there is no assurance that the
filariæ contained in its abdomen came from man; quite as
likely they may come from dog or bird. In such a case one
cannot tell whether the parasite will be digested or will
advance in development. The canine hæmatozoon is digested

By the time this metamorphosis, occupying from four to six days, is completed, the life of the by the mosquito. Therefore it is all-important to work with the proper species of mosquito fed on *human* blood.

I persuaded a Chinaman, in whose blood I had already ascertained that filariæ abounded, to sleep in what is known as a mosquito house in a room where mosquitos were plentiful. After he had gone to bed a light was placed beside him, and the door of the mosquito-house was kept open for half an hour. In this way many mosquitos entered the "house"; the light was then put out, and the door closed. Next morning the walls were covered with an abundant supply of insects with abdomens thoroughly distended. They were then caught below a wine-glass, paralysed by means of a whiff of tobacco smoke, and transferred to small phials having a muslin cover providing for ventilation. As soon as the insects had recovered from the tobacco, and could adhere with their feet to the sides of the bottle, a few drops of water were introduced by means of a pipette. The effect of the tobacco smoke, if it has not been applied too long, is very evanescent, and seems to have no prejudicial influence on the future of the mosquito. From the phials they may be removed from time to time as required, by again paralysing with tobacco, and seizing them by the thorax with a fine forceps. The abdomen is then torn off, placed on a glass slide, and a small cylinder —such as a thin penholder—rolled over it from the anus to the severed thoracic attachment. In this way the contents are safely and efficiently expressed, and observation is not interfered with by the almost opaque integument. If the contents are white and dry, a little water should be added and carefully mixed with the mass, so as to allow of the easy separation of the two large ovisacs. These can be removed in this way with the needle and transferred, if desired, to another slide for separate examination. A thin covering glass should be placed over the residue, which will be found to contain the filariæ either within the walls of the stomach, or, if these have been ruptured by too rough manipulation, floating in the surrounding water. The blood in the stomach

friendly mosquito is concluded; her stomach is empty but for these formidable-looking guests; her ova have been deposited on the surface of the water; her life-cycle is finished, and she dies, probably falling into the water on which her eggs were laid. What now becomes of her guest? As yet we cannot tell for certain. Up to this point the history of the embryo from the time it left its parent in the lymphatic vessel has been followed step by step, and there cannot be the slightest doubt about any part of it. But now an hiatus in our knowledge of its life-cycle occurs; and until some animal, other than man, capable of becoming the host of this parasite is discovered on which we may experiment, or some enthusiast willing to lend himself for the purpose appears, this hiatus is not likely to be filled in except by conjecture—conjecture founded, however, on, and borne out by analogy.

By the time the mosquito dies the parasite has so

of a mosquito that has fed on a filaria-infested man usually contains a much larger proportion of filariæ than does an equal quantity of blood obtained from the same man in the usual way by pricking his finger. Of course the mosquito feeding at night imbibes the blood at a time when it contains the largest number of parasites; but apart from this I believe the insect, or its proboscis, has a selecting faculty probably operating in the way I have indicated in the foot-note at p. 12. Of the large number of filariæ ingested by far the greater part die and are digested, or are expelled in the fæces undeveloped. At the end of the third, fourth, or fifth day, when the stomach is quite empty as far as food is concerned, and an embryo could not easily be over-looked, only from two to six are found in the same or slightly different stages of the metamorphosis I have described.

far advanced in development that there seems nothing
wanting to fit it for independent life and a journey
through the tissues of a human host.   It possesses
an alimentary canal; its head is armed with a
boring apparatus, and it has sufficient strength and
activity to wield this efficiently.   It is also in the
medium most likely to afford it an opportunity of
gaining access to its final host.   What more probable
than that boring its way through the dead and sodden
body of the insect, if it has not already escaped with
the ova, it finds itself in the water, where it will
remain for a longer or shorter time, perhaps to be
captured by some animal in search of food, or, haply,
to be swallowed by man himself? Once in the human
stomach it soon bores its way into the thoracic duct,
or some lymphatic vessel; and working up stream, in
obedience to strange instinct, pierces the lymphatic
glands and finally arrives at its permanent abode in
some distant lymphatic vessel.*   Here it is followed

---

* Helminthology supplies us with many illustrations of
this faculty of travelling towards, and selection of, a suitable
habitat possessed by these lowly-organized animals.   The
same instinct guides the *trichina* to the muscles, the *liver-
fluke* to the gall-ducts, the *giant strongyle* to the pelvis of the
kidney, the *bilharzia hæmatobia* to the veins of the bladder,
the *filaria immitis* to the right ventricle of the dog, the *filaria
sanguinolenta* to his œsophagus, the *filaria corvi torquati* to the
pulmonary artery of the crow, the *filaria picæ mediæ* to the
semilunar valves of the magpie ; and a similar instinct brings
the sexes together in these dark corners.

I would strongly recommend any one desirous of working
at the *filaria sanguinis* of man to make a study of some of the
corresponding parasites of the lower animals.   By doing so
he will not only acquire skill in finding the embryo parasites
in the blood, but will obtain a grasp of the subject which will

by one of the opposite sex obedient to sexual instinct. The couple grow, and for years live together and breed, the progeny passing along the vessels through the glands and into the blood, there to await their

not only interest, but be of great service. The *filaria immitis* of the dog is so common in China and Japan, that workers in these countries can always find plenty of material for study; the examination of a drop of blood obtained by slightly incising or pricking the inside of the ear is an easy method of ascertaining if the animal is filariated. Many birds have hæmatozoa, and in some the parent worms have been found. The common ringed crow of China is usually full of them, and the parent worms can readily be found in the pulmonary artery (p. 24). The magpie of that country is also infested with filariæ, the parents residing coiled up in the pockets of the semilunar valves. The parent worms of the hæmatozoa of the crow and magpie are small and beautifully transparent, and are excellently adapted for showing, under a low power of the microscope, the structures of the filariæ. For examination they should be mounted in a saline solution—urine does very well; if placed in water they swell up and burst, or if in spirit or glycerine they shrivel. The fluid they are mounted in, either for immediate examination, or for permanent specimens, ought to possess a specific gravity approaching that of blood.

For some account of the *filaria immitis* of the dog I would refer the reader to Cobbold's works, or any modern treatise on helminthology; and also to a "Report on Hæmatozoa," by the author, published in the "China Customs Medical Reports" for the half-year ended March 31st, 1877, No. 13. Short accounts of the *filaria picæ mediæ*, of the *filaria corvi torquati*, and of some other hæmatozoa may be found in the "Journal of the Quekett Microscopical Club," vol. vi. 1880. Lewis gives an excellent description of the embryo of a hæmatozoon very common in dogs in Calcutta (the mature form of which has not yet been found, however), in the "Sixth Report of the Sanitary Commissioner for the Government of India," for 1869.

chance of a friendly mosquito to help them, as it had their parents, towards maturity.

This, then, there can be little doubt, is an exact account of the life-cycle of *filaria sanguinis hominis;* and there is nothing in it, or in its relations to the human host, incompatible with the perfect health of the latter. The amount of injury done to the lymphatics by the minute immature parasite in its travels towards its permanent abode is so trifling that no serious disease can possibly result from it. The mature animal itself lies extended in a vessel, and is perfectly adapted by its size and shape for the situation it occupies; it creates no irritation, and the small amount of obstruction it may give rise to is readily compensated for by a rich anastomosis. The embryos move along with the lymph, and being no broader than the corpuscles readily pass the glands, and enter the general circulation. Here they give rise to no trouble, but circulate as easily as the blood-corpuscles.* In fact, the parasite seems in every respect well calculated to live in perfect harmony with its host, and not at all likely to be the cause of serious injury or disease. Nevertheless, that it does become at times a cause of disease and

* Half of the dogs in China, all the magpies, a very large proportion of the crows, and many other birds and beasts harbour similar hæmatozoa, sometimes in prodigious numbers, often hundreds in every drop of blood, and yet their hosts seem perfectly healthy and in no way inconvenienced. The more I learn of these parasites the more I am convinced that when in health, and undisturbed, they are perfectly innocuous. Were it otherwise there would soon be an end to the hosts, and consequently to the parasite itself—both would be exterminated.

danger is certain.   What these diseases are, and
how the parasite brings them about, will appear in
the sequel.

If in a country in which the filaria is endemic (as,
for example, South China) the blood, say of 1,000
natives selected indiscriminately, is examined some
time between sunset and sunrise, in about 100 the
filaria sanguinis hominis will be discovered. If the
history of these filaria-infested individuals is inquired
into it will be found that a considerable proportion
of them enjoy good health; others suffer from
frequent attacks of fever, characterized by well-
marked stages of rigor, pyrexia, and diaphoresis,
resembling in this respect ordinary intermittent fever,
but differing from it in the irregularity and length
of the interval—often weeks or months between
the attacks—and also in the greater length of the
paroxysms; some, in addition to this history of fever,
give a story of lymphangeitis, and may exhibit varicose groin-glands, which, they say, inflame during
the attacks; others have lymph-scrotum; some have
elephantiasis of the scrotum, or leg, or both; others
lymph-scrotum combined with elephantiasis of scrotum,
or leg; one or two may have chyluria; and possibly
there may be a case in which two or more of these
affections are combined. If the 900 in whose blood
no filariæ were found are examined there very probably will not be one, or, at all events, very many
examples of lymph-scrotum, varicose groin-glands,
or chyluria.   There is strong presumption, therefore,
that these diseases and the filaria are somehow
connected.

If we now examine the lymph that has escaped from

a lymph-scrotum, or that has been aspirated from
a varicose groin-gland, or that escapes in the urine
in chyluria,* in the great majority of cases we shall
find in it embryo filariæ. There is a strong presumption, therefore, that the connection between the
parasite and the disease is an intimate one.   If

* The frequent occurrence of red coagula in the urine in
cases of chyluria appears to have had a misleading effect on
the minds of some observers. Such cases have been called
hæmaturia, or hæmato-chyluria. But the presence of the red
and blood-like tint admits of a much simpler explanation
than it could receive did it depend really on blood. It is
unlikely that the embolism of lymphatics which produces the
chyluria should be associated with a disease or lesion of the
blood-vessels causing hæmaturia—two different diseases of the
urinary organs occurring simultaneously in the same individual and not necessarily depending one on the other. It is well
known that lymph as it travels along the lymphatics gradually
advances in development, assuming in the thoracic duct many
of the characters of blood, with corpuscles red and disc-shaped
exactly like those of blood. If in any way the lymph is ob-
structed in its progress towards the blood, there is no reason
for supposing that it should not continue the development it
is known to start on, in normal circumstances, in the lymphatics. Therefore, it happens that the lymph we find in the
urine in chyluria cases has often the red tinge and appearance
of blood. It has lain a long time in the lymphatics and
advanced somewhat in development. The same remarks
apply to the red or dark salmon-coloured lymph that sometimes escapes from a lymph-scrotum. We often find that
the lymph that escapes first on pricking a lymph-scrotum is
milk-like, but after it has run for some time that which
escapes is red and blood-like; in other words, the more
recently formed lymph is colourless, the lymph that has been
formed for some time and which regurgitates from a higher
part of the lymphatics has advanced in development, and is
full of red, disc-shaped corpuscles.

we examine the lymph from one of the cases of lymph-scrotum in which the disease is not associated with filaria in the blood, most probably we shall find the embryo there; and if we amputate such a scrotum we have a good chance of finding in it the parent parasite. We may infer from this that the relation of parasite and disease is one of cause and effect; and, as it would be absurd to suppose the disease the cause of the parasite, we are driven to the conclusion that, in some way, the parasite has brought about the disease, and, inferentially, is also the cause of varicose groin-glands and chyluria.

If we follow up for several years the histories of the cases of lymph-scrotum we shall find that after a time the periodic discharges may cease, and the scrotum gradually assume the characteristic appearance of ordinary elephantiasis. Sometimes we may meet a scrotum in the transition stage, elephantiasis and lymphous discharges co-existing. Occasionally, we find lymph-scrotum and elephantiasis of the leg in the same subject; and in cases of elephantiasis of the scrotum we may elicit a history of previous lymph-scrotum. Further, removal of a lymph-scrotum is sometimes followed by development of elephantiasis of a leg. Once, I have seen amputation of an elephantiasis of the scrotum followed, after many years, by the development of the vesicles characteristic of lymph-scrotum in the operation flaps.* These things

---

For abundant illustrations of these diseases, alone and variously combined, and their connection with the filaria, the reader is referred to chapters ii., iv., and v. of this volume, and to the "China Customs Medical Reports," Nos. 2, 3, 8, 13, 14, 18, and 23; also to an excellent paper by Dr. V. Carter in

occur too frequently to be mere coincidences; and if we reflect that both lymph-scrotum and elephantiasis are diseases of the lymphatics, that they are endemic in the same countries, and affect the same part of the body, we must conclude that they acknowledge the same cause; and this being proved to be the *filaria sanguinis hominis* in lymph-scrotum, it must be the *filaria sanguinis hominis* in elephantiasis.

It has been objected by some that because cases of elephantiasis occur sporadically in countries where the filaria is not endemic, therefore the filaria cannot possibly be the cause in these particular cases, and, inferentially, of those in countries in which the disease is endemic. But in answer to this, it is advanced that the mere presence of the parasite in a man's lymphatics does not necessarily produce the disease; it only does so when it gives rise to obstruction of the vessels, and anything that gives rise to similar obstruction may give rise to elephantiasis. In Europe, where the disease is exceedingly rare, it may be something else; in the tropics, where it is exceedingly common, it is the filaria.

Another objection to the parasite theory is found in the fact that the animal does not always give rise

the "Medico-Chirurgical Transactions," vol. xlv. 1862; and to another paper, by the same author, on "Varix Lymphaticus, its Co-existence with Elephantiasis," in the "Transactions of the Medical and Physical Society of Bombay," 1861, 1862; to Sir Joseph Fayrer's "Clinical Surgery in India;" to "Elephantiasis Orientalis," by Allan Webb, M.D., "Indian Annals of Medical Science," No. 4, April, 1855; and to "Remarks on Varix Lymphaticus or Nævoid Elephantiasis," by Surgeon K. McLeod, A.M., M.D., "Indian Medical Gazette," August 1st, 1874. (See chap. v.)

to elephantiasis, and that the subjects of elephantiasis do not always, or generally, carry the embryos in their blood. How it comes to pass that the animal does not usually give rise to disease has been shown already; how it does give rise to disease in certain cases, and why it is that giving rise to disease the embryos of the parasite do not always appear in the blood, I will now proceed to show.

Lewis, describing the progress of the development of the embryo filaria in the uterus of the parent, says, that the immature animal does not burst its chorional envelope, but that it stretches this, so that after a time, and before it escapes from the vagina of the parent, its shell becomes its sheath. I have not had an opportunity of watching this in the case of the human parasite, but I have frequently watched an identical process in the case of *filaria corvi torquati*, a hæmatozoon inhabiting the pulmonary artery of the common crow of South China. As the embryo nears the vaginal end of the uterine horns by dint of vigorous movements it gradually separates the poles of the ovum; and before it emerges from the parent it has extended them so far that the originally round or oval sac has become converted into a sheath closely applied to the body, the superfluous covering dangling from the head or tail.* Lewis's observation is doubtless correct,

---

* This stretching of the chorion is very easily demonstrated in the parasite I refer to. A crow is selected in whose blood the embryo filaria has been found; the sternum is thrown back, and the heart drawn forward by a hook transfixing the ventricles; the pulmonary vessels are then put on the stretch, and cleared for some distance of lung-tissue by

and is thus fully borne out by analogy. Now, if from some cause or another the embryo *filaria sanguinis hominis* should be hurried into the lymph before the stretching of the chorion commences or is far advanced, what will be the consequence to the human host? In its unextended condition the ovum measures $\frac{1}{500}$-in. $\times$ $\frac{1}{750}$-in., or thereabouts. Its smallest diameter is thus five times greater than that of the fully-formed outstretched embryo we usually encounter in the lymph and blood. It is not too large, however, to pass along the vessels;

scraping with a blunt knife or the handle of the scalpel. The vessels should then be divided as deep in the lungs as possible. As a rule the parent filariæ will protrude from the cut ends, or, if they do not, they can easily be found by slitting up the vessels. Half a dozen are often found together twisted into a sort of rope. A pregnant female—recognized by her large size and plumpness—should be selected,

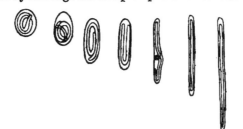

Stretching of chorional envelope by the embryo of *filaria corvi torquati*.

and her body divided at a point a little behind the vulva, which lies within an eighth of an inch of the mouth. Embryos and ova will escape, or can be expressed from the severed uterine tubes. Under the microscope they exhibit the movements I describe—the embryo actively employed in stretching the enclosing bag. By a little searching specimens at all stages, from the spherical ovum to the fully-stretched embryo, can be found.

but when the lymph-stream has carried it to the
glands it is immediately arrested, for there the
afferent vessel breaks up into many very minute
branches which end in the solid parenchyma of
the gland. The imprisoned embryo has no power
to aid its onward progress; but the egg lies like an
embolus, passive, plugging the vessels and damming
up the lymph. There will then be complete stasis
of lymph in this particular vessel as far back as the
first anastomosing lymphatic. Along this the current
will now pass carrying with it other ova; these,
in their turn, will be arrested at the first gland they
reach. And this process of embolism, stasis of lymph,
diversion of current into anastomosis, will go on until
the whole of the lymphatic glands, directly or indirectly connected with the vessel into which the
parent parasite ejects her ova, are rendered impervious,
provided the supply of embolic ova is sufficient, kept
up long enough, or renewed from time to time.

This reads like a piece of sensational pathology,
but I do not describe what I have not seen. On two
different occasions (and from different individuals), I
have obtained the ova of *filaria sanguinis hominis* from
the lymphatics; once from the groin-glands of a case
of lymphatic œdema of the legs,* once in lymph
exuding from a lymph-scrotum.† Cobbold, too, and
possibly Salisbury, have found ova, presumably of the
same parasite, in the urine. The ova obtained from
the case of lymph-scrotum must have come from a
parent on the distal side of the groin-lymphatics.
She must have been miscarrying for some time. The
fact of embryos being found in the blood shows that

* Case XXIV. p. 130.   † Case XXV. p. 131.

they must have had not very long before free access
to it; but as the number of them was very small,
and even these disappeared just before the operation,
embolism of the circle of glands must have been completed. The ova found in the lymph were part of the
crowd effecting this. This worm had lived in the
patient's lymphatics for at least thirty-two years.
When seen he was fifty years of age; his scrotal
disease commenced when he was only eighteen. In
such a lifetime, and in an animal whose reproductive
powers are so active, the chances of some irregularities
in parturition occurring once or oftener must be
considerable. These cases prove, at all events, that
the filaria does at times miscarry. What has happened twice or thrice happens oftener. If we reflect
on the long life of the parasite; the activity of its
generative functions; the exposed position it often
occupies in the legs or scrotum; its liability to
injury, therefore, from mechanical violence; of the
sicknesses of the host, his fevers and blood-poisonings*;
the miscellaneous foods he consumes, some of which
may act on the uterus of the worm as they act on that
of the human subject; we can readily understand how
abortion is brought about. We know the mature
parasite sometimes dies; what kills her, applied in a
less degree, may readily cause her to abort.

* The exanthematous and malarial fevers are well known
to be causes of abortion in the case of the human female. May
they not similarly affect the female filaria? Certain writers,
especially Dr. Allan Webb, maintain very strongly that
syphilis is one of the most common causes of elephantiasis.
May not the explanation of this circumstance (if it is true)
be, that the syphilitic virus operates on the uterus of the
filaria as it is so well known to do on the human uterus?

Of course it is impossible to prove in every case of lymphatic obstruction that this has been brought about by embolic ova. It *must* be a rare thing to see the patient at the proper time; yet, if only once or twice we get the hint of the *modus operandi*, it is readily appreciated and the effects comprehended.

The particular form of lymphatic disease, and the place affected, will depend on the position occupied by the parent worm, on the number of immature ova sho ejects, on the frequency with which these miscarriages are repeated, and on the nature of the tissues involved, and individual peculiarities and accidents.

Let any one with a diagram of the lymphatics before him in imagination locate an aborting female filaria in different situations, and follow out the course her embolic ova would take, and the effect of stasis of lymph, complete or partial, on the different lymphatic areas. If he bears in mind the influence of gravitation, and of inflammation readily induced in tissues whose vessels are congested, he will find that he has got a key to all the elephantoid diseases, and the apparent anomalies in their connection with the filaria.

Suppose we locate her in the lymphatics of the right leg. Her ova will be carried first to the right inguino-femoral glands. After these have been plugged, more or less effectually, anastomosis will carry the ova by the scrotal and neighbouring lymphatics to the inguinal glands of the left side; and when these, in their turn, have been effectually plugged, there must be complete stasis of lymph in both legs and in the scrotum. Perhaps the lymphatics of the latter, overstretched and varicose

from having had to carry the lymph of the right leg
as well as that normally passing through them, give
way; there is then a lymph-scrotum produced, and
in the fluid periodically escaping the young of the
parasite or its ova may be found.   Not having
passed through any glands the lymph will be clear
and straw-coloured as it is at the radicles.   Perhaps
the scrotal lymphatics, being strong and well sup-
ported by a powerful dartos and thick skin, may not
give way; the lymph will then accumulate there, or
gravitation may determine it to a leg, or both legs;
or all of these parts, as not unfrequently happens,
may enlarge.   In such a case, there being little or
no circulation of lymph, probably the parent will
die.

If the worm is located in the scrotum much the
same effects will ensue.   But if she is in a lymphatic
trunk of the pelvis or lumbar region, then, should
the stasis caused by the ova involve the lymphatics of
the kidneys, ureters, or bladder, chyluria may follow.
As the parasite in this case is probably betwixt two
glands, and as the anastomosis of the vessel in
which she lies is guarded in all directions by
glands, it may be impossible, if all of these are
plugged, for embryos to get into the circulation.
Generally, owing to the richness of the anastomosis,
the plugging is not complete, and the parent sur-
vives; on the degree of obstruction, therefore, will
depend the presence or absence of embryos in the
blood.   In addition to producing more or less complete stasis in a particular region, such an accident
among the lumbar or pelvic lymphatics must diminish
the number of vessels available for the transmission

of the lymph from the legs and scrotum. Suppose the
obstruction is on the left side, and is extensive, then
there must ensue regurgitation through unplugged
glands, passage of lymph by anastomosis—either
inside or outside the pelvis—to the right side, where
perhaps alone lymph-paths are open. These are not
sufficient for all the fluid that is formed in those
parts lying below the seat of obstruction. Consequently there is increased pressure in the lymphatics
of the legs and scrotum, and liability to lymph-
scrotum or elephantiasis. Should lymph-scrotum
result, then, as the lymph that escapes must have
regurgitated through several glands, some of them
possibly connected with the alimentary canal, it will
be chylous, or even sanguineous.

When once there is permanent stasis of lymph in
a part, or a lymphorrhagia is established, there is
relief afforded to the remaining lymphatics implicated
in the original area of obstruction; for the amount of
lymph to be transmitted is less by the amount of
that formerly sent from the seat of the developed
elephantiasis or lymph-scrotum. This explains why
excision of a lymph-scrotum is so frequently followed
by elephantiasis of a leg, or by chyluria. The lymph-
scrotum hitherto, up to the time of the operation and
healing of the wound, acted as a sort of safety valve.

The accumulation of a chylous fluid in the tunica
vaginalis, called by Vidal "galactocele," is frequently
associated with filariæ in the fluid and in the blood,
and is explained by the parent parasite being located
in the lymphatics of the cord; or, by these partici-
pating in lymph-stasis produced by obstruction in
glands situated higher up the lymph-circulation. The

double enlargement of the inguinal glands in one-sided elephantiasis is also explained, as is also the so-called metastasis of this disease.

And now my reasons for supposing I would find the parent filaria in the scrotum shown the Society can be understood. The lymph was clear, thin, and straw-coloured, therefore there had been no regurgitation through the inguinal glands; and as no embryos could be found in the blood, therefore, those that appeared in the scrotal lymph must have come from a parent on the distal side of the inguinal glands, possibly in the scrotum.

It is unnecessary to follow out the argument at greater length. Enough has been advanced to show in what way all the phenomena of elephantoid disease may be explained by the theory that the parent parasite is the prime cause, premature birth of the ovum the second, and impaction of the lymphatic glands by the ova the immediate cause.

The impossibility of permanent and thorough cure of elephantiasis is apparent. Much may be done by the knife to remove deformity, and elastic bandaging and other devices for aiding the lymphatics still patent and the blood-vessels to carry off stagnant fluid; but permanent cure of the established disease is impossible.

The prospect on the side of prevention is much more hopeful; for, if people in countries where the filaria is endemic would but cover their wells or water jars with a netting sufficiently fine to keep out the mosquitos, or if they filtered or boiled their drinking water, they would never get the filaria or the disease it produces—elephantiasis.

CHAPTER II.

IT had always seemed strange to me that the *filaria
sanguinis hominis* had escaped observation in the blood
until Lewis found it there in 1872. One would
think there were hundreds of workers in India, and
in different parts of the tropical world, who must have
searched the human blood in the aggregate thousands
of times; yet, notwithstanding this, the parasite,
which in some places is present in every tenth
individual, was overlooked or never found for so
many years. The explanation of this I now offer.
Most workers with the microscope, at all events in
hot climates, pursue their investigations during the
hours when the light is good—that is, during the
day. It will be seen from the following remarks

---

* "China Customs Medical Reports," xxiii. p. 36. We
are indebted to Cobbold for this very apt expression.

that this is the wrong time to search for *filaria san-guinis hominis*.

Two years ago, writing on the habits of *filaria sanguinis hominis*, I remarked that in filarious patients the embryos were frequently temporarily absent from the blood. I was not aware at that time of any law governing this. My examinations were usually made in the early morning, or late in the evening; and of the two assistants I employed, one worked during the day, the other after six o'clock in the evening. I remarked that the former made very few finds in comparison to the latter, but attributed this to accident. Several months ago I gave directions for a filarious patient's blood to be examined daily, and a register to be kept of the examinations. On some days there appeared to be great abundance of filariæ, on other days none, or very few. I noticed that when they were abundant, the examination was made on busy days, when there was much work to be done in the hospital, and extra work of this sort had to be got through in the evening; and that when they were absent, the examination was made during the day. Recollecting the different results obtained by my assistants, according as they worked during the day or after dark, and suspecting now that this was not altogether accident, I made a series of systematic observations every four hours in this patient, and in others, with the view of ascertaining if this periodicity was maintained in every case. I examined a number of patients in this way with the result of finding that unless there is some disturbance, as fever, interfering with the regular physiological rhythm of the body, filaria embryos invariably begin to appear in the circulation at sunset; their numbers gradually increase till about midnight; during the early morning their numbers become fewer by degrees, and by nine or ten o'clock in the forenoon it is a very rare thing to find one in the blood. Till sunset they appear to have completely deserted the circulation; but with the evening they come back again, to disappear in the morning; and so on with the utmost regularity every day, and from day to day. The circle is completed every twenty-four hours, and there are no longer spells of absence, as I at one time supposed, than from morning to evening.

Subjoined is a register of some of the examinations from which I have drawn these conclusions. I have to apologize for the incompleteness of the series of observations in some of the cases; but I often found it very difficult to get a Chinaman to submit during a number of days to the necessary manipulations, and consequently the evidence is fragmentary. But the numbers, taking them together, are quite sufficient to justify my deductions.

TABLE I.

REGISTER OF FILARIA EMBRYOS found in one drop of Blood from the Finger, obtained at the Hours indicated.

Name and Disease.	Date.	A.M.									P.M.											
		4	5	6	7	8	9	10	11	12	1	2	3	4	5	6	7	8	9	10	11	12
Phaia, hospital coolie. Healthy.	1879. July 30					0																
	„ 31					0							0									
	Aug. 1					0												9	8			
	„ 2					0								1	4			24				
	„ 3					0								0								
	„ 4					0												14	5			
	„ 5					0												13	11			
	„ 6					0							0	1								
	„ 7					0								0					16			
	„ 8					0											7					
	„ 9						0															
Tsao, chair coolie. Recent inflammation of cord and testicle.	Aug. 10				0						0									9		
	„ 11			3	0															4		
	„ 12																		8			

Table I.—Register of Filaria Embryos—*Continued.*

Name and Disease.	Date.	A.M.									P.M.											
		4	5	6	7	8	9	10	11	12	1	2	3	4	5	6	7	8	9	10	11	12
Ping, farmer. Healthy.	1879. Aug. 10																	17				
	,, 11					0	0					0						16				
	,, 12											0						28				
	,, 13					0	0					0						14				
	,, 14					2	0							2				6				
	,, 15						2					0	0					4				
	,, 16											0							28			
	,, 17											0							12			
Tso, chair coolie. Elephantoid fever and disease.	July 10													0					28			
	,, 11			6																		
	,, 14				4																	
A gardener. Healthy.	July 15			1		1													13			
	Aug. 10				2							0		0				25				
	,, 11				1													20				
	,, 12																3					

Tchan. Ulcer of leg.																			
Aug. 16									0										4
,, 17		3							0										
,, 18		0							1										
Oah. Elephantiasis scroti and lymph-scrotum.																			
June 16				2			1		:									43	
,, 17	6			1			0		0									24	57
,, 18	23			0			0		0			1	10				37	105	21
,, 19	18			0			0		0									29	
,, 20	15			1			0		1									29	89
,, 21	2			0			0		0									53	41
,, 22	5			0			0		0									17	34
,, 23	23			0			0		0									24	43
,, 24	7			0			0		0									14	
,, 25	14			0			0		0									10	13
,, 26	11			0			:		0									19	
,, 27	5			0			:		0									10	
,, 28	17			0			0		0									12	
,, 29	14			0			:		0									13	
,, 30	14			0			:		0									12	35
July 1	33			1			:		:										

TABLE I.—Register of Filaria Embryos—*Continued.*

Name and Disease.	Date.	A.M.									P.M.											
		4	5	6	7	8	9	10	11	12	1	2	3	4	5	6	7	8	9	10	11	12
Pta. Syphilis....	1879. July 16												0						1			
	" 17			0														0				
Rubbir. Syphilis.	July 20					1								0				5				
	" 21					0								0				0				
	" 22					0								0				1				
	" 23					0								0				0				
	" 24					0								0				2				
	" 25					0								0				12				
	" 26					0								0				2				
	" 27					1								0				0				
Oh. Indurated and varicose groin-glands, and elephanto-oedematous legs.	Aug. 11																		4			
	" 12					0	0					0						4				
	" 13					2						0						5	3			
	" 14						0											4				
	" 15					0							0	0								
	" 16						0					0				0						
	" 17						1					0							18			
	" 18						0					0							5			

Hydro. Fever and hydrocele.

Date																									
June 23				33																0			7		
,, 24				7				0																	
,, 25																		0		0				
,, 26					21			8												0				
,, 27																								
,, 28																								
,, 30				8	18		0		0			0												
July 10				2																				
,, 11				18																				
,, 13				3				0								19		15						
,, 14				5				1								4		0						
,, 15				7				2								3								
,, 16				4				1																
,, 17																		8						
,, 18				4	4													17						
,, 19				10														11						
,, 20				3				1																
,, 21								0																
,, 22																								
,, 24																								
,, 25																								

These figures are abundantly sufficient to establish the diurnal periodicity of the embryo's appearance in the blood. For the meaning of it we have not far to look. The nocturnal habits of *filaria sanguinis hominis* are adapted to the nocturnal habits of the mosquito, its intermediary host; and this is only another of the many wonderful instances of adaptation so constantly met with in Nature.

On establishing this fact these questions occurred to me:—1st. Is the disappearance of the embryos brought about by their death, and have we therefore a fresh swarm every twenty-four hours? 2nd. If they do not die, where do they conceal themselves during the day? 3rd. Has this periodicity any pathological significance?

With regard to the last of these questions I cannot yet give any answer. One could speculate very ingeniously with this for a starting point, but as yet I have no fact of any importance to offer. My conviction is that the pathological significance of *filaria sanguinis hominis* in tropical disease is as yet by no means fully understood, nor the importance of the parasite completely apprehended.

To get an answer to the other two questions, being denied the privilege of post-mortem examinations of men, I turned to the dog, and tried to gain some light from a study of the behaviour of the analogous canine hæmatozoon, *filaria immitis*. First, I endeavoured to ascertain if there is any periodicity of a similar kind observed by the embryos of *filaria immitis*. I examined a number of dogs with this object in view, and the subjoined table is the result :—

TABLE II.

Register of FILARIÆ contained in a drop of Dog's Blood obtained from the Ear at the Hours indicated on successive Days.

BREED	A.M.												P.M.											
	1	2	3	4	5	6	7	8	9	10	11	12	1	2	3	4	5	6	7	8	9	10	11	12
Spaniel	…	…	…	…	174	…	64	…	65	24	44	104	…	210	69	…	…	…	…	683	…	515	…	…
	…	…	…	…	344	…	74	296	112	38	177	18	…	98	131	…	…	…	…	346	…	367	…	…
	…	…	…	…	252	…	178	…	192	42	…	29	…	46	101	…	…	…	…	688	…	…	…	…
	465	…	…	845	…	…	…	…	…	…	…	…	63	…	…	82	253	585	314	354	392	…	…	…
Spaniel	…	…	…	…	8	…	18	…	…	12	8	6	…	22	28	…	…	75	…	58	…	…	…	…
	…	…	…	…	29	…	12	…	…	5	7	6	…	9	19	…	…	98	…	67	…	…	…	…
	49	…	…	41	…	21	…	…	…	…	…	…	7	9	…	35	60	…	…	73	46	39	…	…

TABLE II.—REGISTER OF FILARIÆ—*Continued.*

BREED.	A.M.												P.M.											
	1	2	3	4	5	6	7	8	9	10	11	12	1	2	3	4	5	6	7	8	9	10	11	12
Black and tan terrier.								16	19		9				38		77			48	37 35			
Black and tan terrier.								25	113		22						100				381			
Chinese dog											48				324						1165			
Setter					211 166 304 371 453				162 139 293 164 266				145 162 182 301 324				234 185 215 332				687 614 656 540			

From this it appears that there is a certain periodicity, though not so perfect as in the case of *filaria
sanguinis hominis*. Embryos are never entirely absent
from the blood of infested dogs, though their numbers are always greater during the evening and
night than during the day, the period of greatest
scarcity being from 9 a.m. to 1 p.m. This periodicity has doubtless in the dog, as it certainly has
in man, reference to the habits of the intermediary host. One might express it thus:—As
regards their hæmatozoa, in dogs there is during
the day a remission in numbers, in men an
intermission.

Hoping from a post-mortem examination to get
some information as to what became of the embryos
during the period of remission, I procured a large
Chinese dog, and for a few days made a preliminary
study of the habits of his blood-parasites. But the
brute was so wild, and in such a continual state of
excitement, that the regular remission in the numbers of the embryos was much disturbed, just as
would happen from fever in man. The following is
the register of embryos in a single drop of blood from
the ear, drawn at the hours indicated on successive
days :—

TABLE III.

A.M.												P.M.											
1	2	3	4	5	6	7	8	9	10	11	12	1	2	3	4	5	6	7	8	9	10	11	12
:	:	:	:	:	:	:	28	:	:	:	:	14	:	:	19	:	:	:	:	152	:	:	:
:	:	:	:	:	:	:	:	:	332	217	:	:	280	:	104	:	:	235	:	302	:	:	:
:	:	:	:	:	:	:	254	:	224	:	:	:	452	:	107	:	:	:	202	:	:	:	:
:	:	:	:	:	:	:	225	102	196	:	:	:	:	130	:	:	:	:	:	124	:	:	:
:	:	:	:	:	96	:	:	225	:	:	:	:	:	:	:	526	:	:	:	319	:	:	:
:	:	:	:	35	:	:	:	:	:	:	:	312	:	:	:	509	:	:	167	:	:	:	:
:	:	:	:	98	82	151	:	314	:	:	:	392	:	162	:	:	:	:	:	144	:	:	81
:	:	:	112	:	:	:	:	:	:	:	:	:	:	:	128	:	:	:	:	205	:	:	:

It appeared from this that the embryos were fewest latterly in the early morning. Accordingly I selected one morning at six o'clock, when the embryos in a drop of blood numbered only eighty-two, to administer a dose of prussic acid. The heart was found to contain four female and three male *filariæ immites*. Of the four females three were found to be crowded with embryos at all stages of development, whilst in one the uterine tubes were found to be quite empty, save for a few dead embryos near the vaginal opening and the *débris* of a former pregnancy. In the œsophagus were two large *filaria sanguinolenta* sacs full of parasites, and in the thoracic aorta were many small sacculations and sanguinolenta tumours. Slides of blood or fluid expressed from the following organs — each slide amounting to about one drop — contained embryos in the following numbers :—

Blood from ear before death	82		
„ „ liver after „	324,	365,	204
„ „ lungs „ „	4,582,	1,591,	2,738
„ „ spleen „ „	32		
„ „ kidney „ „	0		

A second dog was killed, strychnine being used instead of prussic acid. Four female and three male filariæ were found in the right ventricle, and in the œsophagus one immature sanguinolenta tumour. Slides of blood gave a very similar result to that obtained in the first dog. No examination of blood before death could be made.

Blood from mesenteric vein after death	123
„ „ lungs „ „	2,631
„ „ liver „ „	53

Blood from portal vein after death   219

   ,,   ,,   kidney   ,,   ,, ...   7

   ,,   ,,   vena cava inferior after death...   270

   ,,   ,,   right ventricle   ,,   ,,   ... 501

   ,,   ,,   spleen   ,,   ,,   ...   0

   ,,   ,,   left external jugular vein   ... 272

Taken in conjunction with the register of embryos free in the blood at different times of the day, I conclude from these figures that the embryos of *filaria immitis* do not die or disappear after a short existence of less than twenty-four hours, but that they rest periodically in the minutest branches of the pulmonary artery; and that when they disappear from the general circulation they are to be found in the lungs. How they manage to maintain their position there against the blood-current I do not certainly know, but I suppose they attach themselves to the inner surface of the vessels in some way, possibly using their oral extremity as a sucker. Occasionally I have seen an embryo thus attach itself to a slide while under examination with the microscope.

I think there can be little doubt that something similar happens in the case of *filaria sanguinis hominis* to what I have shown happening in the case of *filaria immitis*, and that during the period it is temporarily absent from the general circulation it lies resting and waiting for sunset in some of the thoracic or abdominal viscera. What the particular organ is it selects has yet to be ascertained; but this could easily be done by a microscopical examination of the viscera of a filarious subject dying of a non-febrile disease, or suddenly, during the day.

FILARIAL PERIODICITY—*Continued.*

In a former issue of these reports* I pointed out that singular phenomenon in the history of *filaria sanguinis hominis*, which has come to receive the name of *filarial periodicity.* I therein gave part of the evidence on which my assertion of the existence of such a phenomenon was founded; and I ventured to make some suggestions as to its meaning in relation to the life-history of the parasite, and as to what becomes of the animal during its temporary absence from the general circulation. Although the evidence was somewhat fragmentary, yet, taken in connection with a multitude of unsystematic and unrecorded observations, it appeared quite conclusive, at least to my mind. However, in order to elucidate the subject, and render the evidence still more complete, I determined to avail myself of the first suitable opportunity to prosecute systematic observations extending over a period much longer than that of any of the cases recorded in my previous report. Seeing that the periodicity is one of twenty-four hours I thought it possible that it might in some way be influenced, or even caused, by the more or less regular diurnal fluctuations in meteorological conditions dependent on the daily revolution of the earth; or, possibly, that the normal daily rise and fall of body temperature, or other quotidian physiological phenomenon, might have some association with it. I determined, therefore, to add to my observation on the ingress and egress of the embryo parasites others on the temperature and pressure of the

* "China Customs Medical Reports," xxiii. p. 1.

atmosphere, the temperature of the body, and the rapidity of the circulation as indicated by the state of the pulse.

I was able during the summer of 1880 to enlist the services of two sufficiently intelligent lads in every way well suited for my purpose. I trained them to examine the blood, to count the embryo parasites they found therein, to read the thermometers and barometer, and to record all their observations accurately. As they themselves were filarious, and the subject of their own observations, the work could be prosecuted easily, with little fear of interruption, and with the sympathies of the observers entirely on the side of accuracy and truth. Their work I constantly superintended and checked. If error has crept into the chart* into which I have condensed their observations I am certain it is of a trifling and unimportant character, such as is necessarily inseparable from work of the kind; taken as a whole, it may be thoroughly relied on.

Both lads came from Hooihoah, a highly filarious district about three days' journey to the north of Amoy. Li Kha (I. in the chart) was twenty-one years of age, of average size, and in good general health. He gave no history of fever, lymphangeitis, or of any serious disease whatever, and his body appeared to be free from blemish that might be associated with the presence of filariæ. Tiong Seng (II. in the chart), on the contrary, gave a history that distinctly pointed to filarial infection. He, too,

* This chart is reprinted from the "Journal of the Quekett Microscopical Club," vol. vi. 1881.

9

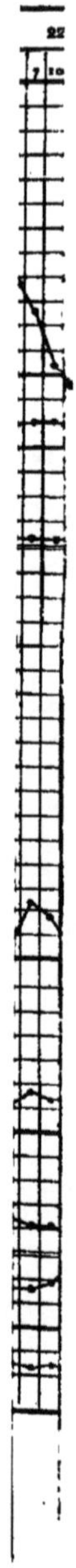
22
7
10

was twenty-one years of age, and in good general condition, but he stated that for six or seven years he had been subject to attacks of what he called ague (lymphatic fever), and that these attacks recurred about once a month. They began, he said, with a feeling of giddiness, and painful aching weariness in the body and limbs. This gradually merged into a cold stage of two or three hours' duration, which was succeeded by a hot stage of very high fever lasting for twenty-four hours and terminating in a moderate diaphoresis continuing for an hour or two. The fever was accompanied by complete anorexia, and during its continuance the inguinal and femoral glands invariably became swollen and excessively painful, those on the right side being more affected than those on the left. With the exception of these attacks, and an orchitis which developed while under observation to be presently alluded to, he never had any trouble about the limbs or genitals, nor other symptom of filarial disease.

The observations by and on these two men I condensed and arranged in Chart I. In explanation of it I may mention that the first three compartments, counting from above downwards, refer to LI KHA (I.); the second three to TIONG SENG (II.); and that the two lowest are occupied by readings of the barometer and ordinary thermometer. At the left hand margin are numbers referring to the filariæ found in a droplet of blood obtained by pricking the finger, and sufficient to occupy in a thin transparent film a slide measuring 1-in. × 1½-in.; also the degrees of temperature of the body, beats of the pulse per minute, temperature of the atmosphere, and baro-

E

metric pressure. Along the top the figures refer to
the date and hour of the day at which the examinations were made.

This chart, recording as it does a long series of
systematic and carefully-made observations, estab-
lishes thoroughly my first assertions about filarial
periodicity. A glance at it shows with what regularity every evening the embryos enter the general
circulation, how they increase in number up to midnight, and how, as morning approaches, they gradually diminish until they completely disappear. Rarely
can one be found from nine a.m. until six p.m., at least
under ordinary circumstances. Since these observations were made I have had the satisfaction of seeing
them confirmed by several others; notably, by Dr.
Myers in Formosa,* and by Dr. Stephen Mackenzie
in London.† Drs. Rennie and Adams of Foochow, I
understand, can also confirm my statements; and I
doubt not that by this time filarial periodicity has
been amply demonstrated by other observers in the
different countries in which the parasite is endemic.

It is a remarkable phenomenon; and now that its
existence is so well established I would commend it
to the physiologist as a possible aid to the explanation of such rhythmical phenomena as sleep, the
evening rise of body - temperature, etc.; to the
pathologist as a possible aid towards the explanation
of diurnal intermission and remission in fevers,
especially of the ague class. Whether it may or
may not be of service in either of these directions it

* "Customs Medical Reports," xxi. 7.

† "Lancet," 1881, ii. 398, 707. "Transactions of the
Pathological Society of London," 1882, vol. xxxiii.

is impossible as yet to say. But though it may lead to nothing in this way, yet the thing itself is so curious and of so striking a character that the mind naturally desires more information about it, and, if possible, an explanation of its object and of its cause.

I have already pointed out* that filarial periodicity is an adaptation of the habits of the filaria to those of the mosquito, the intermediary host indispensable to the future life of the parasite. This is the object of the arrangement; but the particular force or mechanism that operates on the embryo parasite, causing it to appear in the blood normally only at certain hours,—this, the cause of filarial periodicity, has yet to be ascertained. Certain facts, however, have recently been discovered that tend to confine the search to a comparatively limited field.

From the fact that the periodicity is one of twenty-four hours we are justified in inferring that its remote cause is the diurnal revolution of the earth. As affecting the parasite in the human body this may operate in one or two ways: 1st, by means of some of the daily and rhythmical variations it pro-duces in meteorological forces—one or other of these being the direct determining influence that liberates or restrains the parasite; or, 2nd, by inducing in the host of the parasite certain quotidian and rhythmical habits on which, directly or indirectly, the movements of the hæmatozoon depend,—such as the habits of waking and sleeping, exercise, the evening rise of body-temperature, the times of feeding, etc.

* Page 40.

With regard to the first of these, there are at least four principal meteorological phenomena which have a more or less quotidian and rhythmical character, and which one might conceive had an influence in some way on the parasite. These phenomena are —the rise of atmospheric temperature during the day and fall during the night; the decrease of atmospheric pressure during the afternoon; the coming and going of the light; and the diurnal variations in the electrical condition of the earth, as indicated by the magnetic needle. But if we inquire into the behaviour of any of these we shall find that no one of them is so absolutely true in its rhythm as is filarial periodicity. There are frequent exceptions to the general rules that the day is warmer than the night, and that barometric pressure falls during the afternoon. If either of these things, therefore, had anything to do with filarial periodicity, then we should expect to find the latter in entire sympathy with one or other of them, and exhibiting corresponding variations. But if Chart I., in which these are carefully noted, is consulted, it can be seen at a glance how far this is from being the case. The presumption is, therefore, that filarial periodicity is independent of atmospheric pressure and temperature.

To ascertain if the waxing and waning of the light had any influence, I had a filarious subject, in whom I had previously ascertained that periodicity was normal, shut up for several days in a dark room, into which it was impossible for a single ray of sunlight to penetrate. During four days, as far as sunlight was concerned, he was always in the dark, and it was only after sunset that he left his room. A glance at the following table shows that the result of this experiment was entirely negative. I may remark that I was careful not to interfere with his usual habits, and therefore did not disturb him during the night to examine his blood. It was sufficient for my purpose to ascertain approximately the hours of ingress and egress of the embryos, and their conduct during the day.

TABLE showing the NUMBER of EMBRYO FILARIÆ, at the HOURS and DATES indicated, in a SLIDE of BLOOD 1-in. × 1½-in., the SUBJECT of OBSERVATION being kept in a DARK ROOM during the Four Days, November 26th, 27th, 28th, and 29th.

HOUR.	Nov. 24	Nov. 25	Nov. 26*	Nov. 27*	Nov. 28*	Nov. 29*	Nov. 30	Nov. 31	Dec. 1	Dec. 2
7 A.M.	1	4	13	39	25	19	17	16	12	14
11 ,, ...	0	0	1	0	1	0	1	0	0	0
4 P.M.	0	0	1	0	2	0	3	1	2	0
7 ,, ...	5	0	0	0	1	0	5	1	4	0
9 ,, ...	10	8	5	18	10	7	17	18	27	16

* In dark room.

Thus, of the meteorological influences which might be supposed to have an influence on filarial periodicity, three are eliminated. It has been shown that neither temperature, atmospheric pressure, nor light has anything to do with it. There remains only terrestrial magnetism; but, although the rhythm of its variations corresponds very closely with that of filarial periodicity, the progress of discovery within the last few months has rendered a connection between the two so extremely improbable, that I have not considered it worth while to pursue investigation in this direction any longer. It has been pretty conclusively demonstrated that the immediate cause of filarial periodicity is dependent, not on meteorological conditions resulting from the daily revolution of the earth, but on the *habits* this great fact impresses on the human body.

In the "Lancet" of August 27th, 1881, there appeared a letter from Dr. Stephen Mackenzie, in which he announced that a case of chyluria of Indian origin had occurred at the London Hospital, and that the *filaria sanguinis hominis* could be found in abundance in the patient's blood; and, further, that the same periodicity was observed by the parasites in London as had been described as occurring in China. At the meeting of the Pathological Society on October 18th, Dr. Mackenzie exhibited this patient and demonstrated the parasites in his blood; and he also described how he had been able to break up, and even invert periodicity, by simply changing the habits of the patient with regard to the times of sleeping and waking. If the patient slept during the day and kept awake during the night periodicity was inverted. This was a new and important fact. It seemed to be another step towards the explanation of a curious phenomenon; and, impressed by its importance, I took an early opportunity to repeat and vary Dr. Mackenzie's experiments.

The history of the first patient on whom I experimented is briefly as follows :—

CASE I. *Filariæ in the blood; enlarged spleen; anæmia: experiment on inversion of filarial periodicity.*—TIN, male,

aged twenty-five ; Tsongkhæ, Tchangtchiu ; a field labourer.
When twelve or thirteen years old, he says, he had an abscess
in his lungs, which burst, the contents escaping by his
mouth. He spat over a bowlful of blood and pus at the
outset, and continued afterwards for about four months to
cough up similar stuff.* He says the matter expectorated
was thick, viscid, and could be drawn out in a long string ;
the discharge of this was difficult, attended with much
cough ; says he recollects this very well, as his mother used
to slap his back to encourage expectoration. Now he has no
trouble about his lungs beyond a slight cough when he
catches cold. At fifteen or sixteen, had for four months an
eczema on both legs, and at seventeen a very large abscess in
the right popliteal space. Since boyhood has been subject
every autumn to aguish attacks, of a very irregular character,
lasting off and on for about a month every year. Often
during these attacks the inguinal glands, sometimes on the
right side, sometimes on the left side, inflame, but neither
pain nor swelling is ever considerable. Occasionally his
right testicle enlarges without inflammation. These attacks
of fever consist of about one hour of rigor, followed by
three hours of heat and one hour of sweating ; often they
are distinctly tertian, and I think they are genuine ague.
The swelling of the glands does not always accompany the
fever, but the lymphangeitis is usually associated with fever.

He states that some years ago I removed big scrota from
two men living in his village, but he does not know of any
well-marked case of elephantiasis of the leg among his
neighbours. When young he often drank cold water, but
since he became sick he never touches it.

He is very thin, anæmic, and debilitated. An enlarged
spleen extends beyond the border of the ribs. He has no
decided enlargement of glands, scrotum, or legs ; nor does
he give any history of chyluria.

This year his ague began about two months ago. It was

---

* In Dr. Stephen Mackenzie's case, just referred to,
abscess, apparently connected with the thoracic duct and death
of the parent filaria, formed as in this patient.

... in type, and continued in him in a subdued form for about a month. He came to hospital to be treated for his debility, enlarged spleen, and dyspepsia. He took quinine and Flood's pills for a fortnight, and when his health had improved considerably I got his consent to experiment on his ...

From the 10th to the 24th December, 1881, observations were regularly made on this man, the ... quantity of blood ... $\times 1\frac{1}{2}$-in. cover glass) being examined each time. During the first five days sleep was indulged in at the usual hours. Periodic ... having been found normal the time of sleep was changed to the day, and of waking to the night. In December 16th he was not allowed to sleep as ..., but was kept awake ... six in the morning of ... for twenty-four hours. He was ... allowed to sleep all afternoon: and from this ... sleep was always indulged in during the day, while at night he was kept awake. Simultaneously with observations on the number of filariæ present in ... a great quantity of blood, observations on the body-temperature were made in order to avoid the com- ... ever should this occur: but as the ... at the time I have not ... necessary to introduce its record into ... ... this page, on which I have ... ... explanation, I may ... ... refer to the number ... blood 1-in. $\times 1\frac{1}{2}$-in., while ... to the date and hour ... five days the sleeping ... to six a.m. On the sub- ... to the 24th

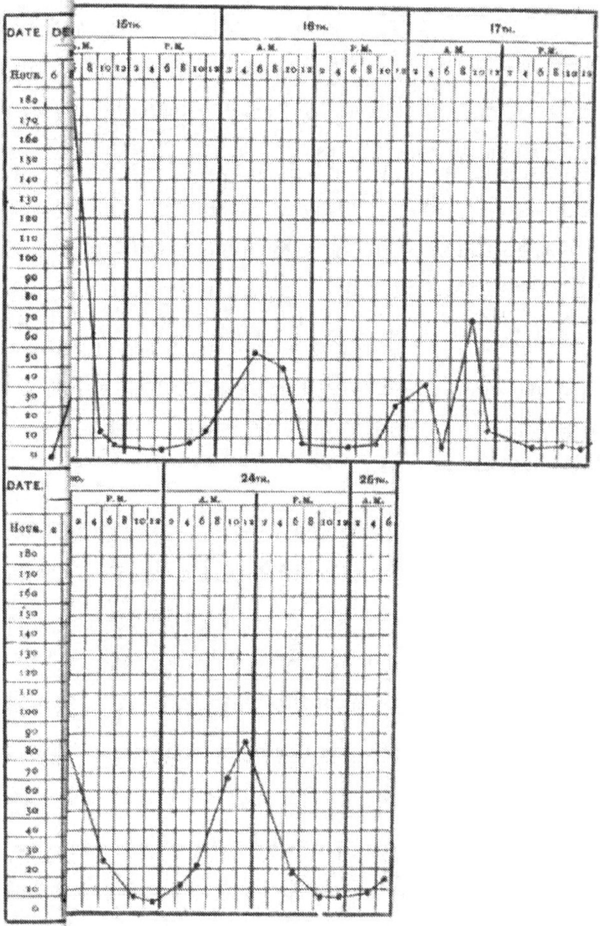
DATE
16TH.
18TH.
17TH.
A.M.
P.M.
HOUR.
DATE.
24TH.
25TH.

tertian in type, and continued on him in a subdued form for about a month. He came to hospital to be treated for his debility, enlarged spleen, and dyspepsia. He took quinine and Blaud's pills for a fortnight, and when his health had improved considerably I got his consent to experiment on his blood-parasites.

From the 9th to the 26th December, 1881, observations were regularly made on this man, the usual quantity of blood (1-in. × 1½-in. cover glass) being examined each time. During the first five days sleep was indulged in at the usual hours. Periodicity having been found normal, the time of sleep was changed to the day, and of waking to the night. On December 14th he was not allowed to sleep as usual, but was kept awake till six in the morning of the 15th—that is, for twenty-four hours. He was then allowed to sleep till afternoon; and from this time sleep was always indulged in during the day, while at night he was kept awake. Simultaneously with observations on the number of filariæ present in a given quantity of blood, observations on the body-temperature were made in order to avoid the complicating effect of fever, should this occur; but as the temperature kept normal all the time I have not considered it necessary to introduce its record into the chart (II., facing this page) on which I have condensed my observations. In explanation, I may mention that the figures at the side refer to the number of filariæ in a slide of blood 1-in. × 1½-in., while the figures along the top refer to the date and hour of examination. For the first five days the sleeping hours were from six p.m. to six a.m. On the subsequent days—that is, from the 15th to the 24th

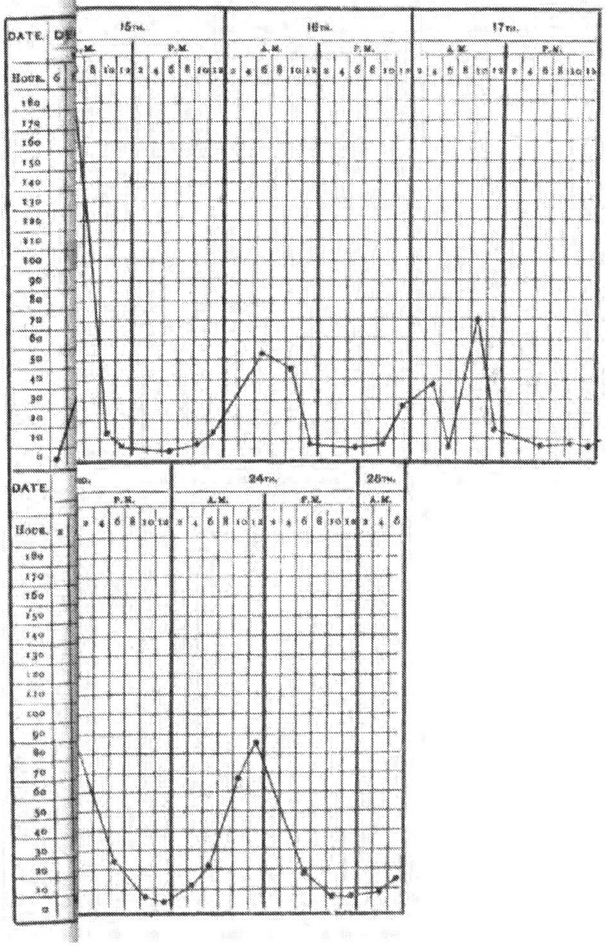
DATE.
15TH.
16TH.
17TH.
A.M.
P.M.
HOUR.
DATE.
24TH.
25TH.
A.M.
P.M.
HOUR.

December—they were from five a.m. to five p.m. During the period when the patient slept at night I did not consider it necessary to wake him at midnight to sample his blood, so in the chart I have assumed that at this hour on these days the filariæ numbered 100. With this exception, only carefully-observed facts are recorded.

It is evident from this chart that Dr. Mackenzie's case was not exceptional; it confirms his statement as to the connection of the sleeping and waking states with filarial periodicity. Something bound up with these states has clearly a powerful influence on the parasite or its young. But, as Dr. Mortimer Granville points out,* it is not simply sleep or waking that has this influence. It is something recurring every twenty-four hours, just as the habits of sleeping and waking recur, and which is capable of being inverted just as these habits are, and by the same means. That sleep does not cause the ingress of embryos is evident from the circumstance that ingress commences hours before the usual time for sleeping, and egress begins hours before the usual time of waking, and periodicity is maintained even though no sleep be indulged in for two or three days, or if sleep is continuous, or nearly so, for as long a time (*see* Charts III. and IV.). The facts of the case seem to indicate that the conditions favourable to the ingress of the parasites become developed ordinarily during the last few hours of the waking state, and that they are slowly eliminated during the last few hours of sleep.

Being anxious to vary Dr. Mackenzie's experiment,

* "Lancet," 1882, i. 314.

and, if possible, obtain additional facts that might aid
in answering the question of the cause of filarial
periodicity, I placed two other men under observation, and variously altered and modified their hours
of sleeping, waking, and eating. Unfortunately, the
man TIN, who was the subject of the observations
recorded in Chart II., had had enough of it, and
seemed very reluctant to submit to a second course of
experiment. I was therefore obliged to fall back on
the two other men, whose stock of filariæ was rather
too limited to show distinctly delicacies of fluctuation.
I give the results for what they are worth. Charts
III. and IV. are arranged on the same plan as Chart
I. The letter " F " is introduced at the hours when
food was taken.

In the case of TIEK Po (Chart III.), the patient slept
from nine p.m. on December 30th to six a.m. on the
31st. From nine p.m. on December 31st to six a.m. on
January 3rd, and from three p.m. on that day to three
p.m. on the 5th, sleep was prolonged by repeated doses of
chloral, the patient being waked up to take food at the usual
hours. From the 5th to the 8th January the sleeping hours
were from nine p.m. to six a.m. Thence until the 20th
sleep was allowed each day from eight a.m. to noon, and
from eight p.m. to midnight. On the 20th-21st the patient
slept from eight p.m. to six a.m., and on the subsequent
nights from nine p.m. to six a.m.

In the case of IN (Chart IV.), sleep was permitted from
nine p.m. on December 30th to six a.m. on the 31st.
The waking state was enforced from this latter hour until
nine p.m. on January 2nd. Thence to January 18th sleep
was enjoyed nightly from nine p.m. to six a.m., and from
nine p.m. on the 18th to noon on the 19th.

The history of the men is briefly as follows :—

CASE II. TIEK Po (Chart III.), male, aged twenty-five ;

AL PERIODICITY.

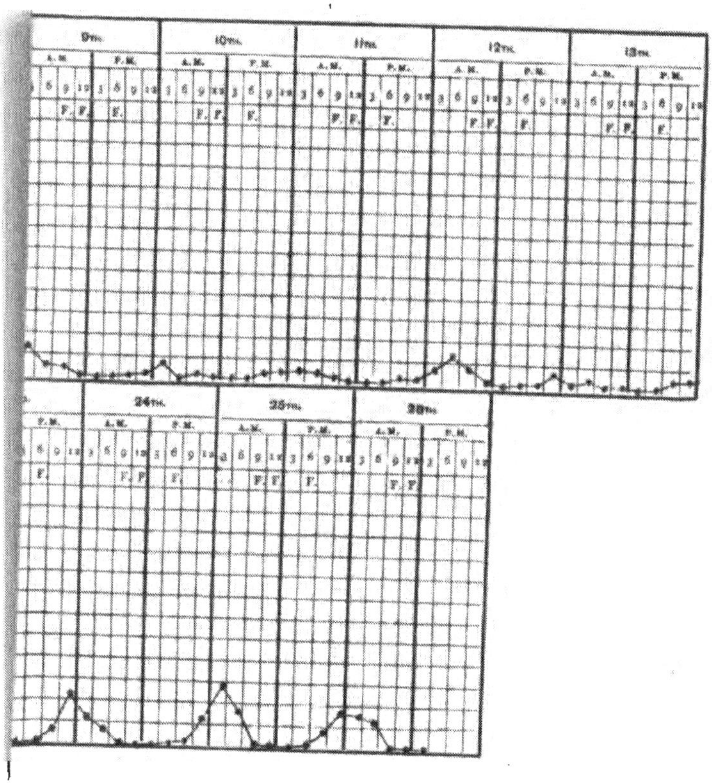
9TH
10TH
11TH
12TH
13TH
24TH
25TH
26TH
A. M.
P. M.
3
6
9
12
F.

Representing the

No. of Embryos in each Slide.
DEC. 30TH
31ST.
JAN. 1ST.
JAN. 10TH.
11TH.
12TH.
A.M.
P.M.

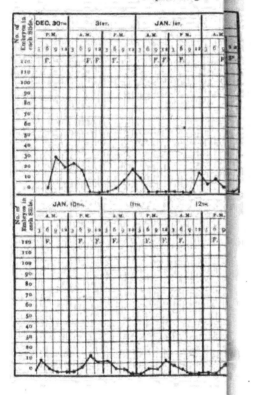

Tchauoi, Tchiupo; farmer. He lives in a village of about 150 inhabitants, and among these are several cases of elephantiasis. Has been ailing for four or five years with ague of tertian type. Off and on has had attacks every winter with the advent of the cold weather. His spleen has been enlarged for several years, and since a year ago he has been subject to attacks of pain and swelling in the left testicle and cord.

On examination his spleen is found to extend to the umbilicus, but no swelling of cord, testicles, scrotum, glands, or legs can be made out; nor is there any history of chyluria or lymphatic fever. Two months ago he had a single fit of fever, and is now very anæmic.

During the time he was under observation he was given quinine and iron in full doses.

CASE III. IN (Chart IV.), male, aged forty-seven; Tang-mng, Tchiupo; farmer. In his village of 200 inhabitants are several cases of elephantiasis of leg or scrotum. One of the latter was operated on at the hospital some time ago. Since boyhood has been subject nearly every year to lymphatic fever of three or four days' duration, associated with swelling of the testicles and scrotum. He has also had attacks of tertian ague and swollen spleen; but at present both spleen and scrotum are normal to all appearance, although the groin-glands are rather large and firm. He says that during his fever attacks these glands swell to the size of fowls' eggs. Had, on admission, right facial paralysis of forty days' standing; this supervened during an attack of fever and delirium. Has never had chyluria nor distinct sign of elephantiasis. His reason for coming to hospital was to be cured of a long-standing chronic ulcer on the left leg. He, too, while under observation, took full doses of iron and quinine.

From these charts we may gather that filarial periodicity is maintained during prolonged watching; and, also, when the hours of eating are changed, so that the middle meal is taken at midnight, and not, as usual, at mid-day; also, that prolonged sleep possibly disturbs periodicity, and diminishes the number of parasites circulating at the time of maximum; and, that when the usual allowance of eight hours' sleep is taken in spells of four hours at a time, at intervals of eight hours, periodicity is disturbed, and the numbers circulating at the time of maximum are sensibly diminished.

When experiments and facts have been multiplied, we may be able to say precisely what is the cause of filarial periodicity. At present, facts are wanting. One which seems to me to have some importance I have not yet alluded to. If reference be made to Chart I., at p. 49, it will be seen that the man TIONG SENG was, shortly after observation commenced, attacked with fever. The fever was consequent on orchitis and lymphangeitis undoubtedly of filarious origin. It will be seen that the body-heat was very high a considerable time before periodicity was affected, and that the usual rhythm of the ingress and egress of the parasites was not renewed for some days after the temperature had fallen to normal. It would seem that the febrile state slowly developed in the blood, or elsewhere, some constituent or condition whose presence or amount influenced the parasites, and that it was not until this pathological product or condition was eliminated or altered that periodicity of a normal character was resumed. May not the waking state, which seems so favourable to the ingress of the parasites, be associated with the development of some physiological condition or product analogous to, or the same as, that resulting in pathological quantity from fever, and the presence of which leads to the presence of the embryo parasites in the blood?

Dr. Mackenzie's discovery has done something to advance this interesting inquiry. He has limited the field in which search need be made. Nevertheless, much has yet to be done, more facts to be collected, before the answer can be given. It seems to me that this will have to be supplied by the physiologist; and when the answer has been given, we shall be in possession of an explanation of many phenomena more important, though not more curious, than filarial periodicity.

CHAPTER III.

ANOTHER point on which I have a few remarks and
facts to offer has recently been discussed by Dr.
Myers in a valuable paper in the twenty-first volume
of "China Customs Medical Reports," viz., the fate
of the embryo parasites which have not been directly
removed from the blood by mosquitos or other means.
Do they, after a brief life of a few hours, die; and
have we to deal with a fresh swarm every twenty-
four hours? Or, do the parasites, after a temporary
appearance in the general circulation, daily retire to
some organ or set of vessels to await the recurrence of
conditions, such as I have been discussing, which
induce them again to circulate? Dr. Myers alleges
that when the blood is examined towards morning,
when the numbers are diminishing, symptoms of
languor are observable in many specimens; and if
these languid individuals are watched for some days
they are found to disintegrate more rapidly than other
and more vigorous specimens obtained during the
earlier part of the night. Dr. Myers's experiments I
repeated many times, but failed to satisfy myself that
what he describes applied to the parasites I observed.
I have kept both morning and evening embryos alive

* "China Customs Medical Reports," xxiii.

on oiled slides for over 100 hours.   In fact, so long
as the serum of the blood remained fluid or viscid, so
long did the parasites live.   I do not think it reason-
able to suppose that animalcules exhibiting such
tenacity of life outside the body should so quickly die
in it, seeing that the circulating blood is their natural
habitat.   But, even supposing that what Dr. Myers
describes is to be found in every case, it does not by
any means follow that this condition of languor is
preliminary to disintegration;   quite as probably it is
preliminary to their passing into some state of rest.
If they died daily in the blood, surely dead specimens
would be frequently met with ; yet so far is this from
being the case that I do not recollect ever to have
seen in freshly-drawn blood a dead filaria—at least,
one whose death could not easily be accounted for by
crushing under the cover glass.   The facts Dr. Myers
adduces are hardly sufficient to found an argument
on.   In a former page* I quoted some experiments on
the destiny of the embryos of *filaria immitis* of the
dog.   Their preponderating abundance in the lungs at
certain times seemed to favour the supposition that
they occasionally retired to the pulmonary circulation,
and I suggested that something analogous might
happen in the case of *filaria sanguinis hominis*.   I
quite agree with Dr. Myers that such evidence is not
conclusive, but analogy must be allowed to have some
weight in inquiries of this nature.   I may mention
here that blood aspirated from the enlarged spleens of
two filarious patients during the day contained no
filariæ ; and that examination of a very small quantity of lung-blood in a case of hæmoptysis, also in a
filarious subject, yielded similarly negative results.

* Pages 45, 46.

If we adopt Dr. Myers's view as to the fate of the embryos, we are driven to the conclusion that filarial periodicity depends on intermittent reproduction, and that a fresh swarm issues from the parent every twenty-four hours. It is possible to put this hypothesis to the test of experiment. In two cases I have had the opportunity of doing so.

I have already* referred to a case of lymph-scrotum in which the parent filaria was found. Prior to operation lymph constantly dripped from ruptured lymphatics on the surface of the scrotum. As there was constant discharge, there was no accumulation. Therefore the lymph that escaped was a fair sample of what was passing the parent worm, and in which she was lying. The lymph was examined three times in one day, viz., at eleven a.m., five p.m., and seven p.m. At each examination many embryos were found. It was evident that the parent was giving birth to them at a time when they are normally absent from the circulation, and that periodicity in this case was independent of the act of parturition. Did filarial periodicity depend on intermittent reproduction, then no embryos could have been found at eleven a.m., and if found at five p.m. they would have been present in the lymph only in very small numbers. I might have made a more extended and careful series of examinations in this case with a view to settle the point, but its importance did not occur to me at the time. Still, as far as they go, these few observations are significant.

Since Dr. Myers informed me of his views I have been on the outlook for a similar or equally suitable case, and some time ago succeeded in finding one which seems to me to settle the point.

* Page 1. See also p. 123, Case XXII.

CASE IV. *Chyluria; filariæ in the blood and urine; an attempt to ascertain whether filarial periodicity be dependent on quotidian and intermitting reproduction, or whether it be altogether independent of the act of parturition.*—IP, male, aged twenty-four; born and residing in Hongsansia—a large village on the North River, about 8 *po* from Amoy; farmer. Never suffered from fever, nor, until lately, from any serious disease. Sometimes has dyspeptic pains in the belly, but nothing of a more serious character. For the past seven or eight years has been troubled with swelling of the left testicle after a hard day's work; the swelling is only slight, and is never accompanied by fever or inflammation.

The chyluria, on account of which he came to hospital, appeared about sixty days before the date of his admission. It began suddenly, after a long, rough, midnight hunt after wild pig on the Hongsan Hills. On his return home he urinated clots, and since then he has constantly, with only one or two exceptions, passed chylous urine. Latterly, he says, the urine has become redder in colour; formerly it was more milky.

He has no elephantiasis or disease of legs, scrotum, or glands; the only thing amiss is slight swelling of the left testicle. Elephantiasis is not common in his village, but there are plenty of cases in the surrounding country. He often drinks cold water.*

---

* The reader will observe that in the record of many of my cases I allude to the drinking of cold water by the subjects of filaria disease. I have been particular on this point, as some have asserted that the Chinese do not drink cold water at all; and that therefore the action of the mosquito as intermediary host of the filaria, and of drinking-water as the medium by which the parasite gains access to the human host, must be a piece of imagination on my part. It is quite true that certain well-to-do and hypochondriacal Chinese avoid cold water, both for internal and external use, but the mass of the people have no such prejudice, at least as regards the internal use; nor, if they had, could they afford to indulge it. Coolies and labourers of all descriptions must drink when thirsty, and they certainly have no time or

The urine, on being passed, is of a dark opaque salmon colour, and reddish clots swim in it. Examined with the microscope it is found to contain many active filariæ, and his blood, if searched after sunset, is seen to be similarly infested.

He complains of much debility and considerable loss of flesh and strength, but his appetite is as good as ever.

As in this case lymph or chyle was nearly always present in the urine, there could be no accumulation in the lymphatics. What at any given time might be selected for examination was a fair specimen of that passing the parent worm; and the presence or absence of embryos in this would be a reliable indication of her activity or repose, as regards the act of parturition. It was therefore a case well suited to settle the question whether filarial reproduction was a more or less constant, or an intermitting process.

The patient was given a placebo, and directed to pass urine into a clean vessel every three hours. The urine thus obtained was well stirred, so as to break up coagula as soon as they formed. An ounce of it was then drawn off into a smaller vessel, and allowed to stand for some hours until subsidence had occurred. A little of the sediment was then taken up with a pipette, one drop of this placed on a suitable slide, and the filariæ it contained carefully counted. Blood drawn at corresponding hours was also examined, and the number of embryos in a slide 1-in. × 1½-in. enumerated. The result of these examinations, extending over one week, I have projected in the accompanying table.

opportunity to boil water on the roads and in the fields, and to wait till it cools before drinking. Boys and girls have none of the hygienic fads that may trouble their seniors, but gratify an appetite regardless of theory or consequence. I have made many inquiries about water drinking among the Chinese, and find that they are very much like other nations in this respect.

TABLE showing the NUMBER of EMBRYO FILARIÆ in a fixed Quantity of BLOOD and URINE, obtained at intervals of Three Hours, from a case of CHYLURIA.*

1881.		HOURS.							
		3 A.M.	6 A.M.	9 A.M.	12 M.	3 P.M.	6 P.M.	9 P.M.	12 MDN.
August 13	Quantity of urine in ounces	...	...	...	12	¼	10	8	12
	Filariæ in urine per slide ..	...	...	...	4	1	10	2	0
	„ blood ditto ..	...	...	...	0	0	0	4	1
„ 14	Quantity of urine in ounces	W 1¾	1	5	5¾	10	W 15	11	W 8
	Filariæ in urine per slide ..	0	4	0	9	1	0	1	0
	„ blood ditto ..	0	0	0	0	0	1	6	8
„ 15	Quantity of urine in ounces	W 4	2¾	¾	6	10	17	16¾	6
	Filariæ in urine per slide ..	2	3	8	17	2	0	11	0
	„ blood ditto ..	2	0	0	0	0	0	12	14

* W before the amount of urine indicates that it was watery and comparatively free from chyle or lymph.

TABLE showing the NUMBER of EMBRYO FILARIÆ, &c.—*Continued.**

1881.	—	HOURS.							
		3 A.M.	6 A.M.	9 A.M.	12 M.	3 P.M.	6 P.M.	9 P.M.	12 MDN.
August 16	Quantity of urine in ounces	5½	W 2½	¼	17½	20	W 22	18½	13
	Filariæ in urine per slide ..	1	0	2	6	3	0	2	1
	,, blood ditto ..	3	0	0	0	0	0	17	11
,, 17	Quantity of urine in ounces	W 2½	W 2	1	6	18	15	6	5
	Filariæ in urine per slide ..	1	0	2	6	6	2	11	2
	,, blood ditto ..	2	0	0	0	0	0	9	7
,, 18	Quantity of urine in ounces	W 8	W 2	3	W 8	16½	11	18½	12
	Filariæ in urine per slide ..	0	0	1	1	11	14	1	0
	,, blood ditto ..	1	0	0	0	0	0	14	9
,, 19	Quantity of urine in ounces	3½	4½	1	..	..	..	..	..
	Filariæ in urine per slide ..	0	0	23	..	..	..	..	..
	,, blood ditto ..	2	0	0	..	..	..	..	..

* W before the amount of urine indicates that it was watery and comparatively free from chyle or lymph.

If these figures are added together, and arranged as follows, the results of this examination become more apparent. It seems to me that they indicate that filariæ embryos are nearly constantly passed into the lymph-stream; and that whenever lymph finds its way into the urine, no matter at what hour, nor how long it has been running, it contains the parasite. Therefore, filarial periodicity is independent of the act of parturition, which is more or less a continuous process.

PRÉCIS of foregoing TABLE.

—	HOURS.							
	3 A.M.	6 A.M.	9 A.M.	12 M.	3 P.M.	6 P.M.	9 P.M.	12 MDN
Total quantity of urine in ounces	25	$14\frac{1}{2}$	11	55	75	90	$78\frac{1}{2}$	56
,, filariæ in a slide of urine	4	7	36	43	24	26	28	3
,, filariæ in a slide of blood	10	0	0	0	0	1	62	50
Average quantity of urine ..	$4\frac{1}{6}$	$2\frac{3}{6}$	$1\frac{5}{6}$	$9\frac{1}{6}$	$12\frac{3}{6}$	15	13	$9\frac{2}{6}$
,, filariæ in a slide of urine	$\frac{4}{6}$	$1\frac{1}{6}$	6	$7\frac{1}{6}$	4	$4\frac{2}{6}$	$4\frac{4}{6}$	$\frac{3}{6}$
,, filariæ in a slide of blood	$1\frac{4}{6}$	0	0	0	0	$\frac{1}{6}$	$10\frac{2}{6}$	$8\frac{2}{6}$
Number of times urine watery	4	3	0	1	0	2	0	1

Although not bearing specially on the subject under discussion, the history of the case after this series of observations was completed is of interest as showing how much mechanical influences have to do in setting up and maintaining elephantoid diseases.

The observations recorded in these tables were completed on August 19th. On the 20th I sent him to bed, and confined him strictly to the recumbent position. Very shortly this had the effect of making the urine in most specimens perfectly limpid. By the end of a week it was permanently clear. He then went home. Six months afterwards I heard of him. He was then quite well, and said he had not passed chylous urine since he left the hospital.

The chyluria was caused in the first instance by the succussion of rough exercise rupturing a congested and dilated lymphatic in the urinary tract; rest, and the removal of lymph-pressure obtained by maintaining the recumbent position, allowed the rupture to heal. The chyluria was thus cured, at least temporarily, and one element in the pathology of these diseases clearly indicated. Chyluria, lymph-scrotum, elephantiasis, diseases caused by lymphatic congestion and varicosity, should be treated on exactly the same principles as diseases resulting from mechanical blood-congestion or venous varicosity. The most important element in the treatment of both forms of congestion is the removal, as far as possible, of fluid pressure, by rest and elevation of the affected part.

CHAPTER IV.*

THE FILARIA SANGUINIS HOMINIS AT AMOY, CHINA;
THE PROPORTION OF THE POPULATION AFFECTED;
THE INFLUENCE OF AGE, SEX, AND OCCUPATION;
THE ASSOCIATED MORBID CONDITIONS.

THE following statistics and observations were made with the view of ascertaining—

1. The degree in which the general population of this district (Amoy) is affected with *filaria sanguinis hominis*.

2. The influence of age, sex, and occupation in determining the presence of the parasite.

3. The morbid conditions, if there are any, with which it is associated.

Before giving the results of my observations, I will premise that, with the exception of elephantiasis and allied diseases, the selection of subjects for examination was made without reference to their physical or social condition. Most were patients at the Chinese Hospital suffering from a variety of miscellaneous diseases, but many were relatives or friends in charge

* " China Customs Medical Reports," 1877, No. xiv.

of patients, and not themselves diseased; others, again, were students at the hospital, or their relatives or acquaintances.

The method of examination I employed was either to divide the droplet of blood, obtained by pricking the finger in the usual way, into six slides; or, what was found to be more expeditious, to transfer the entire droplet to an ordinary slide, using half of another as cover glass. By the latter method the chance of the hæmatozoon escaping from under the cover glass is diminished.

1. *The degree in which the general population of the Amoy district is affected with* FILARIA SANGUINIS HOMINIS.*

Number examined.	Filaria found in	Percentage.	Proportion.†
670	62	9·25	1 in 10·8

* At the time (1876-77) these statistics were collected I had not discovered the law of filarial periodicity; consequently, in order to get an approximate idea as to the prevalence of the filaria in the general population, I had to adopt some plan, such as I describe, of arriving at a fair estimate. I have not had leisure to go over the ground again, but it would be well if some one would undertake this work. Our knowledge of the phenomenon of filarial periodicity would simplify and shorten work very considerably. I may mention that subsequently to the original publication of these statistics they were extended so as to embrace over 1,000 individuals, but the extended series adds nothing of importance to what is here given.

† Dr. J. L. Paterson has arrived at a very similar conclu-

A certain proportion of these cases came to hospital and were examined because they were affected with a filaria disease—elephantiasis. To arrive, therefore, at a correct idea of the degree of infection of the general population, these must not be included in the calculation. Slighter degrees of filaria disease, viz., varicose lymphatic glands and mild cases of lymph-scrotum, do not apply at the hospital on account of these affections, which, as a rule, are discovered only when searched for, the patients coming to be treated for some other complaint. I therefore include all cases of enlarged groin-glands, half the cases of lymph-scrotum, but none of the cases of elephantiasis, as fairly representative of the general population.

A correction must also be made for temporary absence of embryos in the blood in individuals who at another time might be found to possess them. As most of my cases were examined once only, it might so happen that just at the time the examination was made embryos were absent. To arrive at this correction I collected the results of a considerable number of examinations in persons all known to have filaria embryos in their blood at some time, and found from this the proportion of times in which embryos were absent and present. In an aggregate of 89 such examinations they were found 55 times; not found, 34 times. That is to say, if a certain number of persons are examined once for filaria embryos, and these are found in 55 instances, we may infer that they are temporarily absent in a certain number

sion as to the proportion of filaria-infested individuals to the general population in Bahia, Brazil. "Veterinarian," June, 1879.

of others, the proportion of present to temporarily
absent being as 55 to 34.

Number examined, less all the elephantiasis cases and half the lymph-scrotum cases.	Number of cases in which embryos were found, less all the elephantiasis and half the lymph-scrotum cases.	Correction for temporary absence of embryos from the blood.	Total of such cases examined affected with *filaria sanguinis hominis.*	Percentage.
641	51	31·96	82·96	12·81

From these figures we may conclude, that in Amoy
and the surrounding districts, on an average about
one person in every eight is affected with *filaria sanguinis hominis ;* and that in searching for embryos
they will be found about once in every thirteen
persons examined.

2. *The influence of age, sex, and occupation in
determining the presence of the parasite.*

Age.—By classifying the cases according to age,
and in decennial periods, the progressive liability to
filaria as age advances is well demonstrated in the
following table :—

Decennial period.	Number examined.	Filaria found in	Percentage to total cases of Filaria.	Proportion affected.
10 to 20........	35	2	3·22	1 in 17·5
20 ,, 30........	219	17	27·42	1 ,, 12·9
30 ,, 40........	177	16	25·81	1 ,, 11·1
40 ,, 50........	133	12	19·35	1 ,, 11·1
50 ,, 60........	70	8	12·91	1 ,, 8·8
60 ,, 70........	25	4	6·45	1 ,, 6·25
Over 70........	9	3	4·84	1 ,, 3
Not ascertained..	2	..	..	.. ..
Total	670	62	100·00	.. ..

Thus from youth to old age the liability to filaria gradually rises from 1 in 17·5 to 1 in 3. This is to be explained, partly at least, by the fact that the parent worm lives a long time—often a very long time—so that old age not only has its own liability to fresh infection, but possibly inherits the worms of youth and middle age.

Sex.—Owing to the social prejudices of the Chinese, my opportunities of examining females have been few as compared with males—too few to warrant any conclusions as to special liability of a particular sex.

Sex.	Examined.	Filaria found in.	Proportion affected.
Male	620	57	1 in 10·88
Female	50	5	1 in 10
Total	670	62	1 in 10·8

Occupation.—The following table gives the occupations of the different cases examined, and shows the number affected with filaria in each occupation. These are grouped according to social or physical circumstances, as fairly as the nature of the case admits, and proportion and percentage of filaria cases in each group given.

I will attempt no explanation of the figures. They are too few to be of much value. They show, however, that no particular kind of occupation, with perhaps the exception of those of a seafaring character, secures exemption from filaria.

Group.	Occupation.	Number examined.	Total examined.	Filaria found in.	Total Filaria cases.	Proportion affected.	Percentage contributed to total cases.
Rural occupations ..	Cultivators ..	363		24			
	Cowherd	1	365	1	25	1 in 14·6	40·32
	Milkman	1		..			
Trades..	Bakers......	3	..	1			
	Cobbler	1	..	1			
	Cooper	1	..	1			
	Masons......	2	..	1			
	Builders	2	..	1			
	Tailor	1	..	—			
	Saltmaker ..	1	..	—			
	Papermaker	1	..	—			
	Coffinmakers	3	..	—			
	Silversmiths	3	..	—			
	Basketmakers	3	90	—	11	1 in 8·18	17·75
	Penmaker ..	1		—			
	Carpenter ..	1	..	—			
	Reader......	1	..	—			
	Blacksmiths	2	..	—			
	Washerman ..	1	..	—			
	Shoemakers..	2	..	—			
	Sandalmaker	1	..	—			
	Tanner......	1	..	—			
	Pedlars	48	..	3			
	Barbers	10	..	2			
	Tinker......	1	..	1			
Literary	Students	26		2			
	Schoolmasters	6	..	1			
	Doctor	1	..	—			
	Scholars	2	49	—	3	1 in 16·3	4·85
	Artist	1		—			
	Gentleman ..	1	..	—			
	Monk	1	..	—			
	Preachers ..	11	..	—			
Indoor..	Shopkeepers	29	..	7			
	Cooks	6	..	2			
	Shroff	1		1			
	Clerks	4	45	—	10	1 in 4·5	16·12
	Gambler	1		—			
	Dom. servants	4	..	—			
Outdoor	Actor	1	..	—			
	Chair coolies	7	..	4			
	Coolies	20	38	1	8	1 in 4·75	12·90
	Millers......	3		2			
	Soldiers	6	..	—			
	Policeman ..	1	..	1			
Sea	Boatmen	11		—			
	Fishermen ..	4	22	—	—	—	—
	Sailors	7		—			
Occupation unknown..		11	11	—	—	—	—
	Women	50	· 50	5	5	1 in 10	8·06
Total ..	.. .. ..	670	670	62	62	——	100

3. *The morbid conditions, if there are any, with which the parasite is associated.*

No.	Names	Ages.	Sex.	Residence.	Occupation.	Disease, if any.	Duration of disease Years.
1	Augkhi	58	M.	Changchiu	baker	elephantiasis scroti	30
2	Sinto	21	,,	Tinhai	student	none	—
3	Liah	45	F.	Lamoa	farmer	lymph-scrotum	3
4	Kim	33	M.	,,	married	enlarged glands and ulcerated cornea	5
5	Lia	22	,,	Hooiah	chair coolie	enlarged glands	5
6	Tso	50	,,	,,	,,	elephantiasis scroti	15
7	Liengoo	34	,,	Amoy	teacher	fever and anasarca	5
8	Kim	23	F.	,,	spinster	none	—
9	Toon	60	M.	Lamoa	chair coolie	lymph-scrotum	30
10	Nin	26	,,	Lamching	shopkeeper	leprosy	2
11	Beng	22	,,	Petsuia	student	debility	—
12	Boo Biong	38	,,	Chiupo	farmer	enlarged glands	2
13	Lin	27	,,	Oahai	shopkeeper	none	—
14	An	28	,,	,,	cooper	,,	—
15	Leng	30	,,	Lamoa	cobbler	enlarged glands	—
16	Ho	25	,,	Tchoantchiu	farmer	ulcers of leg	5
17	Tscoien	50	,,	Tchiupo	,,	lymph-scrotum	5
18	Thian	43	,,	Thiempo	,,	rheumatism, hydrocele, and enlarged glands	8
19	Tsosim	36	,,	Hooiah	,,	enlarged glands	½
20	Tho	19	,,	Amoy	,,	ague	—

No.	Names.	Ages.	Sex.	Residence.	Occupation.	Disease, if any.	Duration of disease Years.
21	Nug	61	M.	Thiempo	farmer	stricture of oesophagus	¼
22	Khatsin	32	,,	Lamoa	,,	none	—
23	Ngai	36	,,	Tchangtchiu	,,	ague and enlarged spleen	14
24	Le	41	,,	,,	,,	enlarged glands and lymph-scrotum	12
25	Poe	45	,,	Tchoantchin	shopkeeper	elephantiasis scroti	3
26	Phien	70	F.	Ankhoe	widow	heart disease and ulcer	—
27	Simpoo	39	M.	Lantaiboo	farmer	lymph-scrotum	17
28	Tho	40	,,	Tchiupo	,,	chyluria and lymph-scrotum	5
29	What	23	,,	Tchangtchiu	barber	ulcer and enlarged glands	1
30	Ngee	58	,,	Pholam	cotton carder	hydrocele, enlarged glands, and cataract	3
31	Tin	32	,,	Tinhai	farmer	elephantiasis of leg	10
32	Tchian	49	,,	Lamoa	tinker	haematemesis and enlarged glands	7
33	Laang	26	,,	Soasia	farmer	ague, enlarged spleen, and inflamed scrotum	15
34	Kan	72	,,	Amoy	pedlar	lymph-scrotum and chyluria	3
35	Pho	64	,,	Soakoe	shopkeeper	enlarged glands	11
36	Kiong	20	,,	Tangoa	farmer	enlarged glands and cataract	8
37	Tiokna	39	,,	Tchiupo	,,	lymph-scrotum	3
38	Lin	27	,,	Pholam	coolie	ague	—
39	Seng	22	,,	,,	shroff	inflammation of scrotum	1
40	Hoen	27	,,	Tchiupo	farmer	hydrocele	7
41	Hanliong	14	,,	,,	cowherd	enlarged glands and ulcer of cornea	2
42	Tengiee	40	,,	,,	farmer	hydrocele	—

No.	Names	Ages	Sex	Residence	Occupation	Disease, if any.	Duration of disease Years.
43	Sietgoan	37	M.	Tchianan	farmer	enlarged glands and ulcer	4
44	Seng	54	,,	Pholam	,,	lymph-scrotum	14
45	Toon	32	,,	Tohitupo	,,	,,	3
46	Hinlo	48	,,	Ankhoe	cook	hydrocele and fever	—
47	Tanlo	42	,,	Tangoa	mason	lymph-scrotum	19
48	Tanlok	36	,,	Hooioah	barber	,,	13
49	Tantchin	43	,,	Lamoa	cook	,,	13
50	Pong	22	,,	Tchinkang	shopkeeper	hydrocele and enlarged glands	2
51	Ti	48	F.	Tobia	widow	leprosy	—
52	Tchiamtoo	68	M.	Amoy	shopkeeper	enlarged glands and rheumatism	½
53	Heng	25	,,	Taboe	farmer	chronic eczema	—
54	Lin	47	,,	Pholam	pedlar	enlarged glands	4
55	Boon Bor	70	,,	Amoy	rice grinder	internal piles	3
56	Lio	51	,,	Lamoa	farmer	lymph-scrotum and elephantiasis	—
57	Boon Sa	41	,,	Amoy	shopkeeper	none	—
58	Phiet	29	,,	Tchoatng	pedlar	,,	—
59	Ngam	57	F.	Paha	married	enlarged glands and spleen	—
60	Hessi	39	M.	Amoy	builder	none	—
61	Khoan	35	,,	,,	policeman	enlarged glands	—
62	Oon	51	,,	,,	chair coolie	enlarged glands and ulcer of leg	—

A glance at this table shows at once that elephantiasis and allied diseases are much more frequently associated with the parasite than is any other morbid condition. To bring this out more clearly I have arranged the cases as follows :—

		Number examined.	Totals.	Number of Filaria cases.	Total Filaria cases.	Corrected for temporary absence.	Proportion affected.	Percentage contributed.
Elephantoid disease.	Elephantiasis of leg	10	..	1				
	,, scrotum	15	..	4				
	Lymph-scrotum ..	13	..	10				
	Lymph-scrotum and chyluria........	2	} 63	2	} 36	58·25	1 in 1·1	58
	Enlarged and varicose groin-glands	23	..	19				
	Inflamed scrotum and fever	2		2				
	Hydrocele ......}	410	} 412	3	} 16	25·81	1 in 16	25·8
	Other diseases ..}		..	11				
	No disease	195	195	10	10	16·18	1 in 12	16·2
		670	670	62	62	—	——	100

In addition to the statement of the number of cases in which embryos were actually found, I have appended the correction for temporary absence. The propriety of this is questionable, as many cases of elephantoid disease were examined several times before hæmatozoa were found, and as the correction applies only to cases examined once, the addition for correction is too large. I would also add that every patient examined for filaria was not always examined for lymph-scrotum or enlarged glands ; and as these often exist in a slight degree without the patient being aware of it, several such cases have undoubtedly been overlooked, and do not appear under the head of elephantoid disease. The scrotum and glands were carefully examined in every case in which filariæ were found. Making every allowance for these imperfections in the table, it still proves unquestionably the connection between elephantoid disease and *filaria sanguinis hominis.*

CHAPTER V.

CLINICAL EVIDENCE OF THE PARASITIC NATURE OF THE ELEPHANTOID DISEASES.

I PROPOSE in this chapter to bring forward part of the clinical evidence on which the theory of the causation of elephantoid disease by the filaria, as described in the foregoing pages, is founded. The reader will have observed that a principal fact round which the theory has grown is the presence of filaria embryos in the disease I have called lymph-scrotum. This disease is found to be most intimately associated with chyluria on the one hand, and ordinary elephantiasis on the other; so that the three diseases and their varieties may be considered but accidental modifications of the same pathological condition, and etiologically identical. Lymph-scrotum becomes therefore, at all events from a pathological point of view, a very important disease; and a short description of its clinical features may be of use in aiding my readers to recognize and detect it in its milder and more complicated forms. A typical, well-marked case presents no difficulty in diagnosis.

The characteristic feature of lymph-scrotum is the presence on the surface of the scrotum of vesicles and dilated lymphatics, which when they rupture spontaneously, or are pricked, discharge coagulable lymph.

The number and size of these varices differ very much. Perhaps there may be only one or two, perhaps there may be hundreds; and they may be small as millet seeds, or large as the tip of the little finger. Similarly the quantity and physical characters of the fluid they discharge vary between very wide limits. In some cases only a drachm or two of fluid is discharged; in others again five, ten, or fifty ounces will escape; and in several instances the discharge has been so profuse, and has continued so long, that life has been endangered.* In certain cases the discharge is clear and straw-coloured, like hydrocele fluid; in others again it is white, like milk; in others salmon-coloured; and in others again red, like blood; and in the same case variations of colour occur from time to time, and even as the fluid continues dripping from the scrotum. It often happens that the lymph first escaping is milky white, but as it flows it becomes salmon-coloured, and then, finally, before it ceases to flow is red like blood. In every instance the fluid coagulates rapidly and spontaneously, the coagulum contracting rapidly so that after a day or two it may have nearly or entirely disappeared. The fluid then throws down a dark-red sediment, and its surface often becomes covered with a white, greasy-looking pellicle. If the sediment is examined with the microscope corpuscles like those of blood and lymph are found in abundance, and in five cases out of six a careful search is sure to be rewarded with the discovery of many active embryo filariæ.

As a rule in cases of lymph-scrotum, the inguinal and femoral glands are much enlarged. To the touch

* Case **XXV.** p. 131 ; Case **XXII.** p. 123.

they are soft and doughy, and are evidently varicose. If a hypodermic syringe, or hollow needle, is carefully and precisely introduced into one of them, large quantities of lymph exactly like that escaping from the vesicles on the surface of the scrotum can be procured.*   In this also blood and lymph corpuscles

* I would observe, for the information of those who wish to tap the lymphatic glands, that this trifling operation, as far as my experience goes, is unattended with danger. I have done it many times, often many times in the same gland, on the same patient. Within a few seconds of the withdrawal of the needle the neighbourhood of the glands swells suddenly, but by next day all disturbance subsides. Probably the puncture made by the needle in the varicose lymphatic vessels permits the escape of lymph into the connective tissue round the glands, hence the sudden swelling. Bleeding, or profuse escape of lymph, is easily controlled by pressure with the finger. When the glands are very varicose great abundance of lymph may be easily obtained, either by suction with the syringe, or by simply allowing the fluid to percolate through the needle into a glass, the syringe being unscrewed and laid aside altogether. In this way I have many times abstracted several ounces through one puncture at a sitting. When the glands are more solidified, as in advanced elephantiasis, there may frequently be some difficulty in procuring a specimen of lymph; but if the needle is carefully and precisely introduced, and the glands then firmly squeezed between the fingers, the barrel of the needle on withdrawal is found, as a rule, to be full of lymph, and enough for a microscopic examination at all events can be blown out on a glass slide. Occasionally in such a case immediately following the withdrawal of the needle a droplet of clear lymph appears at the puncture, and if one is prepared with a slide may be secured before any sanguineous admixture takes place. When the lymph is very abundant large numbers of filariæ may be found by collecting in a conical glass an ounce or two of the fluid, and waiting till the coagulum, which

and, usually, filaria embryos abound.   Pressure with the palm of the hand disperses the swellings, but on removal of the pressure the glands rapidly refill. Occasionally a case of lymph-scrotum is met with in which the glands are not involved ; and, conversely, cases of varicose groin-glands are to be found in which the lymphatics of the scrotum are not dilated.

If a lymph-scrotum is amputated, and before the operation wound is sewn up pressure is made on the dilated inguino-femoral glands, lymph, often in great abundance, can be made to regurgitate from dilated lymphatic vessels on the upper and femoral side of the exposed spermatic cords.

A notable and characteristic feature of lymph-scrotum, as it is of ordinary elephantiasis, is the frequent occurrence of an erysipelatoid inflammation of the affected parts, accompanied with a species of fever which Sir Joseph Fayrer has very aptly called " elephantoid fever."   This fever is ushered in with severe rigor, and is thus often called ague ;   the hot stage is prolonged, and may be associated with delirium ; after a day or two it ends in diaphoresis, and not uncommonly an escape of lymph from the

presently forms, has dissolved, and a dark brown sediment of corpuscles collected at the bottom of the glass.   This process of coagulation and solution usually takes from twenty-four to thirty-six hours.   In the sediment living filariæ are always very abundant, and can be found readily.   Of course, in employing the needle of the hypodermic syringe in this way one must be sure of the diagnosis, and that there is no hernia ; regard also must be paid to the femoral artery and the large veins in the neighbourhood.   With a little caution and skill no danger need be apprehended.

scrotum. There is no regularity in the recurrence of the attacks of scrotal inflammation and fever.* Very often abscess forms in the affected tissues, and until the pus escapes attacks of inflammation and fever are of frequent occurrence. Often it is an attack of scrotal inflammation and fever that first calls the patient's attention to his disease. These attacks are readily induced by exposure to cold and wet, by the friction of the thighs against the scrotum in walking, by slight injury, and by alcoholic or other excesses.

It is very singular that a disease of so striking and peculiar a character has received so little attention from observers. Though many cases of lymphorrhagia from different parts of the body, especially from the legs and groins, have been published, and although in descriptions by various authors of cases of elephantiasis lymphous discharges from the parts affected have been alluded to, yet the first description of lymph-scrotum as a distinct pathological condition dates so recently as 1854. It was reported by Mr. Ardaseer Jamsetjee, in the "Transactions of the

* Some writers maintain that the recurrence of the attacks of elephantoid fever bears a certain relation to the lunar cycle. I have often inquired about this from my patients, but never succeeded in establishing any proof of such a relationship. The common causes of inflammation in other parts of the body are the common causes of elephantoid inflammation and fever; and injuries of any sort, prolonged exercise, dependent position of the affected parts, attacks of malarial fever, and so forth, more readily cause inflammation in parts suffering already from lymphatic congestion or obstruction. There is nothing *specific*, however, in the fever or in the inflammation.

Medical and Physical Society of Bombay" (vol. ii. new series, p. 341), as follows :—

"Patient, a stout Parsee merchant, aged fifty; duration of the disease, seventeen and a half years; preceded by an injury. There are vesicles of a minute size at the front and upper part of the scrotum, where the integument is rough and thick; from this a milky white fluid exudes, sometimes to a large amount; this coagulates, and afterwards separates into two parts; there are no (?) corpuscles in it. The discharge is irregular in its appearance, and subsequently the vesicles subside. The general health is good. The author supposes the occurrence of this discharge prevents increase of the hypertrophy of the scrotum which otherwise might take place."

This is the case as condensed by Dr. Carter; he adds that the character of the "milky" discharge was not detected.

A second and a third case were published in the "Edinburgh Medical Journal" for January, 1860, under the title of "Milky Exudation from the Scrotum," as an extract from the "Report of the Missionary Hospital at Kumleefou in the Western Suburbs of Canton, for the year 1858-59," by Wong Fun, M.D. The description of the first of these is accurate and careful, and corresponds with many of the cases I have observed.

The next and most important notices are by Dr. Vandyke Carter in the "Transactions of the Medical and Physical Society of Bombay," 1861 and 1862, and in the "Medico-Chirurgical Transactions" (vol. xlv. 1862). In these publications will be found several well-marked cases very fully and carefully described, along with an elaborate discussion on the pathology of the disease, and its connection with the ordinary form of elephantiasis.

In his work on " Clinical Surgery in India," published in 1866, Sir Joseph Fayrer describes a case on
which he operated—he calls it " nævoid elephantiasis."
He again alludes to the disease in his " Clinical and
Pathological Observations in India," published in
1873, and also in the " Practitioner" for August,
1875.

A paper by Surgeon K. McLeod in the " Indian
Medical Gazette," for August, 1874, contains an interesting analysis of the literature of this subject, and
describes a well-marked case observed by the writer
himself.   He calls the disease " varix lymphaticus,"
and remarks that it is not of unfrequent occurrence
in India.

These notices, along with brief allusions to it by
Dr. Druitt in the " Medical Times and Gazette,"
by Dr. Lewis in papers in the " Reports of the Sanitary Commissioners with the Government in India,"
by Rindfleisch, by Paget (" Lectures on Surgical
Pathology," third edition), and numerous cases published by myself in the " China Customs Medical
Reports," included nearly all that had been written
on this subject up to 1875.   Since that date the
literature of lymph-scrotum has considerably expanded, but it is still a little known disease.

What I have written, however, is sufficient to give
the reader an idea of what lymph-scrotum is ; and
will prepare him to understand better what is meant
by this term in the narrative of the cases I will now
give illustrating the connections between this disease,
chyluria, elephantiasis, and the other filaria diseases.
These cases bear out what I have already stated, that
the various combinations and transitions of these

diseases one into another prove the identity of their pathology. It is true that in fully-developed elephantiasis the filaria is by no means constantly present; but if we can show that elephantiasis is only a modification of such diseases as lymph-scrotum and chyluria, in which the filaria is almost invariably found, we have strong reason, in addition to that derivable from other considerations, for deciding that true elephantiasis is also a filaria disease.

I propose to arrange and narrate these cases in the following order :—

1. Cases of chyluria in which the *filaria sanguinis hominis* was found.

2. Cases of lymph-scrotum in which the *filaria sanguinis hominis* was found.

3. Cases in which chyluria and lymph-scrotum were combined or alternated.

4. Cases showing lymph-scrotum passing into elephantiasis scroti, the diseases co-existing.

5. Case in which lymph-scrotum followed an operation for elephantiasis scroti.

6. Case of elephantiasis of the leg following operation for lymph-scrotum.

7. Cases of lymph-scrotum and elephantiasis of the leg combined.

8. Case of lymphorrhagia in an elephantoid leg, combined with varicose groin-glands and filariæ; chyluria subsequently developed.

1. *Cases of chyluria in which the* FILARIA SANGUINIS HOMINIS *was found.*

The number of times in which the parasite has been found in cases of chyluria is now so great, that the almost invariable association of the parasite with this disease is considered established. It is, therefore, unnecessary for me to narrate any cases specially under this head. It will suffice if I refer the reader to those detailed by Lewis ("Reports of the Sanitary Commissioner with the Government in India," No. 6, 1869); to the remarkable case narrated by Dr. Stephen Mackenzie in the "Transactions of the Pathological Society" for 1882, vol. xxxiii.; to the cases of Wucherer in which the parasite was first found; and to several given by myself in this volume, and in different numbers of the "China Customs Medical Reports." It may be safely affirmed, that in five cases out of six of chyluria in which the parasite has been carefully and properly searched for it has been found, both in blood and urine. But to be found, the parasite must be searched for at the proper times and in the proper way. It is useless to look for it in blood drawn during the day; it must be drawn at night, and best between the hours of nine p.m. and three a.m. If looked for betwixt these hours, and in these cases, it will almost invariably be found. In the urine it is as abundant during the day as during the night; but it will not suffice to examine a drop only of the urine. A considerable quantity should be collected, well stirred so as to break up all clots, and then stood for several hours, during which the filariæ it may contain will subside to the bottom of the vessel. The sediment ought then to be removed by a pipette, and carefully searched with the microscope. In this way the parasite will nearly certainly be found.*

* Many fail to find the embryos because they use glasses of too high a magnifying power. A half-inch or three-quarters object glass is quite high enough for searching

The occasional absence of the embryo in cases of tropical chyluria is readily accounted for by the death of the parent worm, an event that does sometimes happen.   But, although the original cause of the disease has disappeared, it does not follow that the damaged lymphatics recover.   An acquired varix of any sort does not tend towards recovery.   Consequently chyluria may not always be coincident with the presence of the worm in blood or urine, and yet the original cause of the disease was the worm.

2. *Cases of lymph-scrotum in which the* FILARIA SANGUINIS HOMINIS *was found.*

The same remarks apply to lymph-scrotum that apply to chyluria.   In five cases out of six the filaria is present in blood and lymph, and, by observing the precautions as to time and method of search, can readily be found.   Many cases of filarious lymph-scrotum are now on record, so that it is hardly necessary for me to do more than give a brief sketch here of one or two by way of illustration.

I should premise that the cases I record were seen and examined by myself at the Chinese Hospital in Amoy.   In some instances the patients were only seen once; in others, again, they remained a considerable time under observation, so that the record is not in every case equally complete.

CASE V. *Lymph-scrotum ; filaria embryos in blood and lymph.*—MNG, male, aged thirty-seven, a farmer from Tchoantchiu, Lamtia; on a visit to Amoy.   In his village (population over

---

purposes.   A large field by using these low powers can be examined quickly and thoroughly.   It is perfectly useless to attempt finding the embryos with an eighth, or a quarter even.

2,000) he knows of three other cases like his own, he says, but does not know of any cases of elephantiasis. The water he drinks comes from a stream; it is stored in a jar which is filled up every day, but emptied and cleaned only every four or five days. Sometimes he drinks water from the paddy fields.

When young (about fourteen years of age) had fever, and since then, whenever his work lies in the wet rice fields, has frequent attacks of fever; of late, for the last three or four years, the attacks have been very frequent. The attack sometimes comes on while he is in the field, sometimes later when he is in bed. It begins with a severe rigor, lasting for about two hours; then he has high fever for twelve hours; and then the attack terminates in a short and mild diaphoresis. The scrotum and inguino-femoral glands become swollen and very painful during the hot stage of the fever, and it is not until after three days that he can leave his bed, the scrotum beginning about that time to discharge. He has been subject to these discharges for two years only. The glands have been enlarged for seven years, but he has been subject to fever for over twenty years. The fever has been of the same (elephantoid) character from the beginning—never of the tertian or quartan ague type. He has never had chyluria.

His lymph-scrotum and enlarged inguino-femoral glands are typically developed. He has no elephantiasis. He is thin, but looks in good health.

April 27th, 1880.—I drew off from the inguinal glands with a hollow needle specimens of lymph as follows:—

From right side 2¼ ounces pale salmon-coloured and coagulating, at 6.30 a.m. This specimen I marked "1."

From left side 2 ounces dark salmon-coloured and coagulating, at seven a.m.; marked "2."

From the right side, at mid-day 1¾ ounces salmon-coloured and coagulating; marked "3."

From the left side at the same time 2 drachms dark salmon-coloured and coagulating; marked "4."

From the right side at six p.m. 1½ ounces pale salmon-coloured and coagulating; marked "5."

Blood drawn from the finger at seven a.m. contained in one slide measuring 1½-in. × 1-in. five filariæ; a similar quantity drawn at mid-day contained no filariæ; at 5.30 p.m. no filariæ; at seven p.m. one large drop contained eight filariæ.

The lymph drawn off from the glands was allowed to stand that the coagulum might have time to contract or disappear; on April 28th—next day—various glasses were examined.

Six a.m.—No. 1. Still contains a slight coagulum; filariæ abundant. No. 2. Dark red, fibrous, semi-coagulated deposit; four filariæ in one slide. Nos. 3, 4, 5, still contain large coagula.

Six p.m.—No. 5. Still coagulum; no filariæ found in two large slides. No. 4. Two dead filariæ in one slide. No. 3. No filariæ in one slide examined. No. 1. Two slides examined; one filaria. No. 2. No filariæ in one slide.

April 29th, six a.m.—No. 1. One slide; no filariæ. No. 2. One slide; four living active filariæ. No. 4. No filariæ in one slide. No. 3. One living filaria in one slide. No. 5. No filariæ in one slide.

April 30th.—Drew off from right inguinal glands about two ounces of clear, straw-coloured, coagulating lymph about 11.30 a.m. After the coagulum had disappeared and the glass containing the lymph had stood for some hours, large numbers of filariæ were found in the sediment.

The next case is an example of ordinary lymph-scrotum. I introduce it here partly as being an example of the presence of the filaria in the blood and lymph, and partly as it records an experiment on the effect of chloroform narcosis on filarial periodicity. In this instance the chloroform had no effect in throwing the embryos into the general circulation at a time when they are normally absent; but in the second instance of a similar experiment, to be presently narrated, it apparently did have some effect (see p. 104).

CASE VI.   *Lymph-scrotum; removal under chloroform;
periodicity of filaria embryos not affected by the chloroform.*
—Lo, male, aged thirty-six; a merchant in Amoy. This
was a case of ordinary lymph-scrotum, with filariæ both in
blood and lymph.

August 11th, 1880.—The scrotum was removed under
chloroform. The operation lasted from 12.30 to 1 p.m.
During its progress blood was drawn from a finger three
times and examined with the microscope, but no filariæ were
found; and immediately prior to the operation, also, it was
ascertained that they were absent from the blood. Blood was
again examined at three p.m., when the effects of the
chloroform had passed off, but embryos were still absent.
Filaria embryos in very small numbers were found in the
juices expressed by the contracting scrotum after removal;
but though carefully searched for during two hours no parent
worm was found in the tumour. The blood was frequently
examined during the subsequent progress of the case, viz.,
on August 25th, September 10th, 15th, 24th, and October
10th, and was on each occasion found to contain filariæ; of
course the examinations were not made during the day.

CASE VII.   *Excessive development of lymph-scrotum and
varicose inguinal glands; filariæ in scrotal lymph* (see plate IV.).
—HOCK SENG, male, aged thirty-two; born in Tchoantchiu,
but been in Amoy, where he works as a tailor, for the last
sixteen years. He was brought up in very poor circumstances, and has been delicate since childhood, being subject
to attacks of quartan ague.

I saw him on August 9th, 1881. He told me his scrotal
disease began about three years before with fever and local
inflammation, and pain over the bladder. Since then the
groin-glands and scrotal lymphatics have become varicose.
Lymphous discharge from the scrotum occurs every few days;
sometimes only once a fortnight. When once started it continues for two or three days. On first appearing the discharge
resembles rice-water, but as the flow continues it gradually
becomes sanguineous. Fever is now very irregular, and is
always accompanied by much pain in the groins, scrotum, and

belly.   He told me that a long transverse scar in the left groin over Poupart's ligament was the result of a large abscess he had five or six years ago.   There is a small reducible swelling which may, or may not, be a hernia on the left side; he says its appearance was coincident with the development of the scrotal disease.   The groin-glands on both sides, but especially the left, are very large and soft.   The scrotum is dusky, thickened, large, and pendulous; its lower part is like a soft elephantiasis, but on both sides, and also behind and in front, the lymphatics are exceedingly varicose; in front and behind they are like bunches of purple grapes, on the sides they are smaller—like currants.   A small incision into one of the varices gave vent to a large stream of dark brown, blood-like lymph.   The stream was large and strong, as if from a big vein.   Fearing to injure him by drawing off too much, to stop the flow I had to take up the wound with a forceps and include it in a ligature.   He told me the scrotum had discharged only four days before.   He distinctly states that, as a rule, under ordinary circumstances of spontaneous rupture, the discharge at first is white, like pus, and then as it runs becomes gradually dark red, resembling what I drew off. I found three filariæ in a small drop of lymph drawn at seven p.m.

Many cases similar to these, as regards the presence of embryo filariæ in blood and lymph, I have recorded in the "Customs Gazette." It is unnecessary, therefore, to multiply examples here.

3. *Cases in which chyluria and lymph-scrotum were combined or alternated.*

The first example recorded of this combination we owe to Dr. Vandyke Carter; but as at the time the record was made the filaria had not been discovered, no mention of its presence was made.   Probably had it been looked for in the proper way it would have been found.   Describing the case, Dr. Carter says:—

"Four months since, the scrotum began to enlarge; native

applications were made, and it was only after a time that the peculiar corrugation of the skin appeared. The milky discharge regularly occurs spontaneously, and it intermits; at present it has been going on for two days, and he reckons to have lost about one pound of fluid daily. It does not issue from any one spot, but from several ; it may be according to the number and position of the tubercles that have burst. When it ceases, and sometimes also when the discharge is going on, the urine becomes chylous, and frequently coagulates. Such is his own account. Health indifferent. No appetite. He was afterwards admitted into hospital, and I found that the tumefaction of the inguinal glands seemed to alternate with the appearance of chyle in the urine. This circumstance was sufficiently established. The parts became tumefied a short time (two or three hours) after a full meal, and then again subsided. There did not appear to be any regularity in the appearance or disappearance of chyle in the urine."

Lewis records a case in which the scrotum became the subject of elephantoid enlargement (probably lymph-scrotum) two years after the appearance of a filarious chyluria. Towards the end of 1873, the same observer had the opportunity of examining a case in which chyluria was combined with an elephantoid state of the scrotum. Filariæ were found.

"The patient was a Jew, and was suffering from acute pain produced by an inflamed condition of a moderately large scrotal tumour. This tumour had been coming on for many years, and increased and diminished in bulk at irregular intervals. It was studded with tubercular prominences, soft and yielding to the touch, and when a trocar was introduced several ounces of sanguineous fluid were withdrawn . . . . . . The chyluria had only been observed about a fortnight previously."

He also mentions a third case which supplied

specimens of the filaria, and in which an elephantoid condition of the scrotum and foot co-existed with chyluria.*

The following are examples of the combination occurring in my own practice :—

CASE VIII. *History of elephantoid fever; chyluria and lymph-scrotum co-existing; elephantiasis of the scrotum.*— KUGHOK, aged twenty-five; a labourer from Chin Chiu, in very poor circumstances. When sixteen years old he had what he calls fever and ague, which lasted for four days, and during this time his scrotum got inflamed and swollen. When the fever was past the inflammation and swelling subsided. From that time till he was seen at the hospital he had fever attacks twenty or thirty times a year, his inguinal glands and scrotum enlarging, the latter gradually becoming covered with small vesicles which on bursting would discharge about twelve ounces of milky fluid. On admission he was seen to be strong and well-built, and, with the exception of slight anæmia, had the appearance of a man in the enjoyment of good health. He stated that he had been passing "white" urine for some weeks past. On examining the scrotum it was found to be much enlarged, the skin thick and coarse, the penis almost completely buried, presenting in fact the usual appearances of an elephantiased scrotum of about two pounds weight, with, in addition, numerous transparent vesicles covering the surface. On puncturing one of the vesicles about ten ounces of fluid were discharged, the first portion being clear, like water, then gradually becoming like milk, and the last few ounces like a mixture of blood and milk. On the following day his urine, which was chylous before, became natural. The scrotum was amputated; it weighed two pounds, and had the usual appearance of

---

* In this connection the reader is referred to a remarkable case related by Roberts in his " Urinary and Renal Diseases," in which a varicose condition of the lymphatics of the abdominal integument was associated with chyluria.

elephantiasis, a strong outer rind enclosing a blubbery-like mass. The filaria was not searched for.

CASE IX. *Elephantoid fever; lymph-scrotum and intermitting chyluria.* — TANHOK, aged twenty-six; a labourer from Chiupo, in poor circumstances, and of a phthisical family. When ten years old he had fever and ague, which lasted for thirty days. When twenty - three had a second attack of fever, this time accompanied by pain and swelling of the inguinal glands and scrotum. After about three weeks, and when the fever had subsided, the scrotum became covered with numerous small vesicles, which caused much annoyance by constant itching. After ten months a vesicle burst, discharging a considerable quantity of white fluid. From that time, sometimes once in five days, sometimes once in ten or twenty days, a vesicle would burst discharging ten to fifteen ounces of fluid. On coming to hospital he was suffering much from anæmia and debility, but his appetite and digestion were unusually good. A vesicle was cut open, and fluid, at first white and afterwards of a reddish-white colour, continued to be discharged until the afternoon of the following day. The fluid measured fifty-four ounces, not including some few ounces which were unavoidably lost. Four days afterwards he had a second discharge of fluid—twelve ounces—from the same vesicle as we had opened. A week afterwards the patient called attention to his urine, which, he said, he had been unable to pass for eight or ten hours. The urine was in large quantity, of a reddish-white colour, and coagulated rapidly. He complained of pain in the passage. After a few days the urine again became natural. The diseased part of the scrotum was removed by the knife, and the parts healed up rapidly, but on the day following the operation the urine became white, like milk. After three weeks he returned home. Two months afterwards he again came to hospital. He stated that his urine was still white, although at times it was almost natural. A small patch—about an inch square—of the skin of the scrotum was seen to be covered with vesicles. It was excised. While he remained in hospital he continued to pass from seventy to eighty ounces of chylous urine daily, of a specific gravity of about 1015. Though the filaria was searched for in this case it was not found, probably because at that time the habits of the parasite were not known, and the proper methods were not employed.

CASE X. *Hæmatozoa; chyluria and lymph-scrotum.*—THO, aged forty, a farmer from Tchiupo, Pholam-Kio. Says there is no elephantiasis or leprosy among his neighbours. Till thirty-five or thirty-six years of age he was a strong, healthy man, but about that time had, from what I can make out from his description, prolapsus ani. When eighteen years old had an abscess in his scrotum. Elephantoid fever began about his thirty-sixth year; the attacks consisted of rigors, pyrexia, and sweating, the whole paroxysm lasting about six hours. Glands and scrotum have been affected since this fever first showed itself; their periodical swelling and inflammation appearing, from his description, to be secondary to the attacks of fever. These attacks occur irregularly from once to several times a month; the last attack, only four days prior to his admission to hospital. He knows of no cause for his complaint.

His is a fine specimen of lymph-scrotum; it has never discharged spontaneously, but on pricking one of the many vesicles on its surface two to three ounces of rapidly-coagulating straw-coloured lymph exudes. There is no hardening, and but slight enlargement of the scrotum, which is soft, silky, and pendulous. The inguinal and femoral glands of the left side are very much enlarged and varicose; those of the right side are also enlarged, but to a less extent, and are harder to the touch.

Three months ago he first noticed blood and clots in his urine; at the time he had a slight attack of the usual fever. Since that time his urine has never been quite free from blood and clots, the amount of these diminishing or increasing according to the amount of work he does. Since the establishment of the chyluria fever attacks are more frequent, and he has become very anæmic and debilitated; so much so that he cannot keep on his legs for any length of time, but is compelled to lie or sit down.

July 11th, 1877, he came to hospital; on the 14th I note that his blood and chylous urine had been frequently examined (during the day), but in neither had filariæ been found. He was put on large doses of gallic acid and tonic doses of quinine. On July 15th I note that I examined two specimens of his urine. One of them, passed during the previous night, had been standing in a conical glass for about twelve hours, and had separated into three well-marked zones; the uppermost, and most bulky, was of a pale salmon colour; the middle was of a considerably redder tinge than the former; and the lowest was of a dark red, like blood, and formed a mere sediment at the bottom of the vessel. I examined many slides of this sediment, and, after a prolonged search, found one dead hæmatozoon in it. The other specimen of urine, passed only two hours before examination, was a dirty red colour throughout, with several very firm clots floating in it; specific gravity, 1012. No filariæ were found in it. Blood, lymph, and oil corpuscles abounded in both specimens of urine.

July 16th.—An assistant found two filariæ in blood to-day.

July 19th.—He found one filaria in blood last night, and this morning I confirmed his observation by finding two more.

July 22nd.—He returned home, having derived no benefit from the very large doses of gallic acid he had been taking.

CASE XI. *Hæmatozoa; chyluria and lymph-scrotum.*—KAU, aged seventy-two; a pedlar living in Amoy. He says that there is no elephantiasis in his family; that about thirty years ago he visited Formosa and Tientsin, but with this exception has always resided in and about Amoy. Thirty or forty years ago had an aguish attack of very short duration, and, as far as his memory serves him, had abscess in the scrotum about the same time. It was not, however, until a few years ago that he became liable to attacks of swelling of the groin-glands; this recurred every three or four months. His scrotum has been swollen, a little over two years only. Occasionally he has rigor and fever, and then the scrotum itches excessively, inflames, and becomes covered with minute white vesicles; these burst and discharge a large quantity of fluid. When this happens he passes urine; white like milk, for a few days; when the discharge from the scrotum ceases, that of chyle in the urine also disappears. This chyluria has occurred many times during the last two or three years. He is much troubled with rheumatism.

The scrotum is large, pendulous, and vesiculated, and the glands on both sides are swollen and varicose.

Filariæ were found in great abundance in his blood. Doubtless they were present also in scrotal lymph and chylous urine, but I have no record of their having been searched for.

4. *Cases showing lymph-scrotum passing into elephantiasis scroti, the diseases co-existing.*

When we inquire into the early history of cases of ordinary elephantiasis of the scrotum, in many instances we get a description of lymph-scrotum; and are often told that when the discharge characteristic of this affection ceased to recur, the scrotum began to enlarge. I have operated on over a hundred cases of elephantiasis of the scrotum, large and small, and the early history of many of these was that of lymph-scrotum. Dr. Allan Webb, in a paper on "Elephantiasis Orientalis" in the "Indian Annals of Medical Science" (No. 4, April, 1855), details such a case. His patient gave the usual history of fever and inflammation.

"After each attack of fever, during a period of four years, the scrotum would transude a quantity of white, ropy-looking matter, which very much reduced its bulk. . . . But about ten months ago this suddenly ceased, and the tumour rapidly doubled in size. The manner of transudation, he says, is that during the paroxysm of the fever minute vesicles, about the size of a pin's head, appear; they are scattered all over the surface of the tumefied scrotum; they become very prominent and distended with serum (?) after the fever subsides, and break rapidly and discharge their contents."

When these periodical escapes of fluid ceased to recur, then the tumour assumed gradually the bulk and appearance of ordinary elephantiasis. I have recorded several examples of scrota in the transition state, and. possess notes of many more. It will suffice if I give three or four by way of illustration.

CASE XII. *Hæmatozoa; elephantiasis and lymph-scrotum combined.*—ANG KHI, aged fifty-eight; a cake baker from Changchiu, in comfortable circumstances. He states that when twenty-eight years of age, in the spring of the year he had an attack of what he calls ague, accompanied by inflammation of the scrotum. The fever lasted for only one day, but it was two months before the scrotum returned to its original size; before doing so it desquamated. Since that time he has had attacks of fever every year from four to eight times, each attack being accompanied by inflammation of the scrotum. Two years ago the scrotum did not, as formerly, recover after the fever, but remained swollen, and has grown steadily ever since. Formerly he was stout and strong, but for the last ten years has lost flesh. He has never had chyluria. His scrotum presents the usual appearance of elephantiasis. I suppose it to weigh about eight pounds. On its under surface there is a solitary vesicle, about the size of a split pea, and near this a bunch of dilated lymphatics; pricking any of these gives vent to a drachm or two of coagulating milky lymph. His blood, on examination, was found to contain many filariæ.

. CASE XIII. *Hæmatozoa; lymph-scrotum and elephantiasis scroti.*—POE, aged forty-five; a shopkeeper from Tchoanchiu, Tchin Kang. No leprosy or elephantiasis in his family, but a neighbour has elephantiasis of a leg. He states that at seventeen he had a tertian ague, lasting for two months. At forty-two had his first attack of the fever, which for the last three years has never left him for more than a few days at a time. Describes the fever as commencing with a feeling as if produced by retraction of the spermatic cords, giving rise to so much pain that he has to leave off work at once; this is immediately followed by rigors, fever, and sweating, the whole attack lasting about six hours. He says that his disease commenced by an attack of chills coming on in the middle of a very long and wet journey; when he got home he had fever, and next day he discovered that his groin-glands were enlarged, and his scrotum œdematous; in a month's time vesicles had formed on the surface of the scrotum. With successive attacks of fever the scrotum inflamed, became permanently enlarged, and at times discharged a white lymph in great abundance, four or five ounces. His fever, he says, never comes on during the night.

A mass of elephantiasis, weighing about two and a half pounds, involving both penis and scrotum, was removed, and the penis and testes were left bare to cicatrize. This process took about four months to accomplish; during the whole of that time he had no recurrence of the fever, which, prior to the operation, attacked him every few days. The glands in the left groin appear to be quite healthy; not so those on the right side, where a large tumour is formed by the enlargement of a bunch of them over the saphenous opening, and another cluster over Poupart's ligament. To the touch they are firm, and not varicose. Hæmatozoa were found in his blood.

CASE XIV. *Elephantiasis of scrotum and lymph-scrotum combined; filaria embryos in lymph from varicose groin-glands, but not in the blood.*—HENG, aged thirty-eight; a chair coolie from Hoöieoah. He says there is no case of elephantiasis in his family or neighbourhood, as far as he knows. Has had an enlarged scrotum for three or four years, which he attributes to his having slept on one occasion on the hillside in the rain. Has six or seven attacks of elephantoid fever every year, accompanied by the usual and characteristic inflammation of the scrotum. Last year there was a discharge from the scrotum, but there had been no recurrence of the discharge since then. When admitted to hospital the scrotum had rather the appearance of elephantiasis, although it felt softer than is usual in a well-marked case of this disease. No distinct dilated lymphatic was visible on the scrotum, but the inguinal and femoral glands on both sides were much enlarged, some of these being varicose, others consolidated. He said he never had chyluria.

I thrust the needle of a subcutaneous syringe into one of the varicose inguinal glands, and in this way procured a small quantity of milky lymph. In this I found a languid filaria embryo. The following morning I examined six large slides of this man's blood, equal to about six droplets, but could find no filariæ in it. The subcutaneous syringe was again used to extract lymph from the groin-glands. In the clear lymph thus obtained four filariæ were found in six slides, one slide containing two. The embryos were very languid in their movements, one at least being shrivelled, the lash at its head standing out very distinctly, even when viewed with a low power. Besides the unquestionable filaria embryos, numbers of threads, about $\frac{1}{100}$-in. in length, were found in the lymph, their appearance suggesting the idea that they were the collapsed sheath of the embryo, the body of which had disappeared by absorption or disintegration.

This man's scrotum was amputated. It had the appearances usually met with in ordinary elephantiasis, and weighed about two and a half pounds. Though carefully dissected no mature filaria was found. After the operation the swelling of the glands subsided, and the case did well. Though examined daily for nearly a month no embryo was ever found in his blood.

CASE XV. *Lymph-scrotum passing into elephantiasis; hæmatozoa in blood and lymph from scrotum; amputation.*— POA, aged forty-one; a farmer from Tchin Kang, Lamoa. At eighteen or nineteen had shivering and fever, with bleeding from the nose and general dropsy. This dropsy, he says, lasted for about a month, and then everywhere disappeared but in the scrotum, which remained red and thickened. Often since that time he has had attacks of elephantoid fever and, frequently, discharges from his scrotum.

There is no positive history of chyluria, but he said that before the first attack of scrotal swelling he passed white urine in small quantities.

The scrotum is very large for an ordinary lymph-scrotum; it is greater than a large pumelo, and is dense. Inguinal and femoral glands on both sides prominent and varicose. There was a copious discharge of milky-red coagulating lymph from a small wound on the penis, accidentally made whilst clipping hair prior to operation.

October 8th, 1880.—A slide of blood, 1½-in. × 1-in., drawn at 6.15 p.m., contained eleven embryos. About an ounce of lymph collected and set aside. Lymph had been running all day, and that set aside for examination was collected about six p.m.

October 9th, six p.m.—Many dead embryos found in the dark red lymph-sediment.

October 10th.—Scrotum removed under chloroform at noon to-day. The operation and narcosis lasted about twenty minutes. The scrotum and foreskin weighed four pounds and a half. Specimens of blood drawn at the time of the operation were examined for filariæ, with this result :—

Blood from finger before operation ... ... no filariæ.
   ,,   ,,   ,, after ,, ... 4 ,,
   ,,   ,, spouting artery during operation ... 6 ,,
   ,,   ,, incision in penis ,,   ,, ... 1 ,,

At six p.m. a specimen from the finger contained twenty-seven filariæ.

October 15th, slide of blood at 5.30 p.m. ... 1 filaria
  ,, 16th   ,,   ,, 5.30 a.m. ... 5 filariæ
  ,, 22nd   ,,   ,, 5 p.m. ... 8 ,,
November 3rd ,,   ,, 5 p.m. ... 7 ,,
The case did well.

The chloroform in this case, unlike what happened in one already narrated, apparently had some effect in throwing the embryo filariæ into the general circulation at a time when they are normally absent.

CASE **XVI**. *Lympho-elephantoid scrotum ; filariæ in lymph from scrotum and in the blood.*—THI EN IET, aged forty-eight; a farmer from Tchiupo. None of his relatives have elephantiasis, but the disease is very common in his neighbourhood. He says that he often drinks cold water in the warm weather; it comes from a well, but is usually stored in a jar for two or three days; there are many mosquitos in his house, and they can easily get access to his water-jar. Until his scrotal disease began had no disease but ague. His scrotum has been affected for over ten years. It began with inflammation and elephantoid fever. The first attack kept him in bed for over a month, and until he was relieved by a copious yellow, serous-looking discharge from the surface of the scrotum. Since that time has had many such attacks irregularly once or twice a month, but the discharge is independent now of the fever, and occurs very frequently. Rough trousers by scratching are sufficient to induce it, and it will run for an hour at a time. He has never had chyluria.

The scrotum is as large as his head. It is rough, thick and in a state of genuine elephantiasis, with a dense rind apparently about an inch in thickness. The penis is quite buried in the mass. In fact, but for three or four large vesicles the size of swan shot, and which on being pricked discharge a sanguineous lymph, it is an ordinary example of elephantiasis. The groin-glands are slightly, but only slightly, enlarged, and are not at all varicose. Two ounces of a reddish sanguinolent lymph distilled *guttatim* from a vesicle in about a quarter of an hour. On the surface of the scrotum are several small tumours resembling in size and shape the vesicles, only differing from them in being solid; evidently at one time they had been vesicles, but had solidified; others again were semi-fluctuating, apparently in a transition state.

November 28th, 1880.—In scrotal lymph, drawn at 6.30 p.m., I found many filariæ. Blood drawn at the same time contained eight to a slide $1\frac{1}{2}$-in. × 1-in. At 8.30 p.m. the lymph continuing to run had become clearer and was free from red tinge. Three drops of it were searched and only yielded two filariæ. The blood now contained twenty-three to the slide.

November 29th.—Scrotum amputated. It weighed four and a half pounds. Several filariæ were found in lymph from a vesicle, but at the same hour (mid-day) none could be found in the blood.

January 2nd, 1881.—The case has done well. Every night till date the blood has been examined, about nine p.m., and on every occasion was found to contain filariæ.

I could give many more examples of lymph-scrotum passing into elephantiasis. It is quite a common thing where filaria disease is endemic; but the opposite or converse phenomenon of elephantiasis terminating in lymph-scrotum is very rare indeed. I have only met with it once; the following are some notes of the case.

5. *Case in which lymph-scrotum followed operation for elephantiasis scroti.*

CASE XVII.—ONG AN, aged thirty-five; a field labourer from Tchoantchiu. Came to hospital in 1872 to be operated on for elephantiasis of the scrotum. His disease began about five years before. He gave the usual history of elephantoid fever, inflammation of the scrotum, and gradual enlargement of the tumour. He was operated on, and a tumour weighing ten pounds was removed. In 1879 he came to see me—that is seven or eight years after the operation. He said that after leaving the hospital he went home with his wound quite healed, and returned to his fields working hard as an ordinary labourer. For five years his scrotum gave him no trouble whatever, but kept sound and free from inflammation or swelling of any sort; and in other respects he enjoyed good health. About this time, however, he had a mild attack of elephantoid fever; and since then, especially after unusual exertion, has had many similar attacks—about five or six, he says, every year. The fever is not accompanied by distinct inflammation of the scrotum, but this swells and feels painfully constricted. Sometimes, about three times a year, but only for the last three years, he has a discharge of milky coagulating fluid from the scrotum. When the discharge begins to flow it is clear, like water, but after running for five or six hours it gradually becomes opaque and milky, and continuing for about six hours longer it gradually ceases to flow. He is quite positive in his statement that he never had any sort of lymphorrhagia before the operation, and neither before nor since has he had chyluria.

I carefully inspected his genitals and found them, as far as the operation was concerned, in a very satisfactory condition, nearly free from elephantoid thickening, and with the flaps freely movable over the testicles. The right flap is the larger, and just at its most dependent part there is a circle, an inch and a half in diameter, of slightly elephantiased tissue. The cicatrix and penis are quite sound. Nearly over the whole of the scrotum, especially at the lower and back part, are scattered at wide intervals minute vesicles, milky-white, and no larger than pins' heads. They are arranged singly, in irregular groups, and in short beaded lines. One of these vesicles I opened, and procured in a very short time a large quantity of milky-white coagulating fluid of the usual lymph-scrotum character. Perhaps in half an hour I collected two ounces. The inguinal and femoral glands of the left side are large and solid; those of the right side are nearly normal.

I examined his blood carefully four times betwixt six p.m. and nine p.m., but it contained no filariæ; neither could I find any in the sediment of three ounces of scrotal lymph.

The gradual passage of lymph-scrotum into elephantiasis can easily be understood, but this supervention of lymph-scrotum on elephantiasis is not so easily explained. I assume that the lymphatics carrying the lymph from the apparently sound operation flaps were damaged before the date of the operation, but only slightly so; that gradually they are becoming more occluded from contraction at the seat of the original obstruction, and are now no longer capable of transmitting the entire production of lymph by the tissues. When the obstruction has become complete, and should the accumulating lymph not be discharged from the surface of the scrotum at short intervals, this man will certainly have a recurrence of his elephantiasis.

6. *Elephantiasis of the leg following operation for lymph-scrotum.*

I can imagine no stronger proof that elephantiasis and lymph-scrotum are but varieties of the same disease, than is supplied by this case. When the lymph-scrotum, or, in other words, the tissue permitting the escape of lymph, was removed by an operation, elephantiasis, or, in other words, complete stasis and organization of lymph, began.

CASE XVIII. *Lymph-scrotum and elephantiasis of the scrotum combined; filariæ in lymph and blood; operation; elephantiasis of leg developed* (see Plate V.).—OAH, aged nineteen; a rice pounder from Khoan Kau, E-ong. No relatives, as far as he knows, affected with elephantiasis. E-ong is a small hamlet with about 100 inhabitants in the suburbs of Khoan Kau. The people drink well-water, which they store in large jars; it is often kept for several days, no particular attention being paid to keeping the jars covered or clean. When sixteen or seventeen years of age the patient was frequently laid up with attacks of an evanescent fever, accompanied by a relapsing inflammation (it may have been of the testicle) in the right side of the scrotum, and enlargement of the right and left groin-glands, more particularly of the right. When fifteen he had an abscess in the left groin (scar is visible still), and another the same year in the right leg near the ankle; at the time the whole leg was swollen (describes it as "toa kha tang," or "big heavy leg," the expression for elephantiasis). The swelling remained for about one month, but subsided on the

bursting of an abscess, and now no thickening remains. The
scrotal inflammation and the fever recurred about twenty
times each year, but it was not until about a year ago that
the scrotum discharged. When this happened it occurred
daily for some time, and then dried up for about three
months; but for three or four months hardly a day has
passed without an escape of lymph. When he came for the
first time to the hospital there had been no discharge for
several hours. A vesicle was pricked, and from then till
the time these notes were made—four days—it has dripped
constantly. In one hour I saw collected two ounces of a
milky coagulating lymph.

Four days subsequent to his admission to hospital I
examined the scrotum carefully. He had it trussed up in
a headcloth, on removing which a fine stream of lymph was
forcibly projected by the contraction of the dartos, as if by
a syringe, from a minute orifice at the lower part of the
scrotum. Half an ounce ran in a fine capillary stream in
the course of a couple of minutes. The scrotum was as
large as an average pumelo. The skin of the penis was
found to be distinctly elephantiased; and the skin visibly
and palpably thickened over both groins, the lower two
inches of the abdominal wall, and over Scarpa's triangle on
both sides. The upper and thigh surfaces of the scrotum
were covered by a fine, silky skin, freely movable over the
thickened substratum; a little lower down the skin was
thickened and adherent, as in elephantiasis; lower still small
ampullæ were visible; lower down these became larger, and
along the raphe they were the size of small beans. Pricking
any of these vesicles the usual fluid escaped. This was most
distinctly a combination of elephantiasis and lymph-scrotum.
The groin-glands were large, but they did not feel varicose;
however, on piercing a gland on the right side abundance of
straw-coloured lymph was procured; in this fluid I found
filariæ. I examined the lymph which dropped from the
scrotum, and also blood from a finger, and in both of these
found filaria embryos. During the short time required to
make this note more than three ounces of fluid distilled from
his scrotum. In a few ounces of this fluid a feeble coagulum

formed, which, in the course of eight or ten hours, contracted to about one-sixth the bulk of the fluid. The clot was then tough and fibrous. A small portion was removed, and placed between two glass slides, and firmly pressed out; in the fluid thus expressed, surrounding and within the open meshes of the fibrine, were many living specimens of the filaria. I found none in the serum the clot floated in. It would appear, therefore, that the coagulating fibrine caught the filariæ, and, contracting, carried them as in a net, thus concentrating them in the clot. Some of the filariæ were very robust and active; others again were languid, spotted, and shrivelled looking. In one such atrophied specimen the lash was quite visible with a low power, as were also many short fibres about $\frac{1}{100}$-in. in length. Twelve hours afterwards the coagulum had completely disappeared; a flocculent sediment lay at the bottom of the glass, and in this great numbers of filariæ were found.

I removed this scrotum. Shortly after the operation the diseased tissues were found to weigh about a pound and a half. During the operation there was considerable bleeding, and also an escape of lymph from two dilated lymphatics, one on either side, just external to the spermatic cords. Firm pressure with the palm of the hand caused lymph to well up in great plenty from these dilated vessels. This man was kept under observation for upwards of two months. The wound healed soundly, and the swelling of the glands decreased. His blood was examined daily, and during several days six times in the twenty-four hours; but, unless the examination was made during the day, it was invariably found to contain embryos (see register, p. 37). Mosquitos were also fed on his blood, and the embryos ingested by these insects were found to undergo the metamorphosis I describe (p. 13), confirming thereby observations made on several previous occasions. The mosquitos and scrotum were sent to Dr. Spencer Cobbold, and have been frequently examined by competent men in London.

The diagnosis of lymph-scrotum passing into elephantiasis, subsequently, in this case, received singular and unquestionable confirmation. The man returned to hospital with his right leg, the flaps left at the operation, the cicatrix, and the integuments of the lower part of the abdomen, all in a typical state of elephantiasis. He stated that he had kept quite well for four months after leaving me (that is for six months after the operation), and was able to resume his rather fatiguing work of rice pounding. He was then attacked with elephantoid fever, and pain in the right groin, and sometimes had a discharge of straw-coloured fluid from the operation cicatrix, and also from the thickened skin over the right groin and thigh. As he is covered with itch, it is probable that this discharge was provoked by scratching. Three months ago the right leg inflamed and swelled up to a great size, and since then he has had three attacks of this inflammation, accompanied by elephantoid fever. He says he had also a large swelling at one time on the upper and inner surface of the left arm, which threatened to suppurate; but, after troubling him for ten or twelve days, it disappeared spontaneously. The skin of the flaps and the cicatrix are rough, hard, and tuberculated, as in elephantiasis of some standing; the skin over the abdomen and groins is coarse, and evidently considerably thickened; while the swelling of the thigh and leg is best described as brawny, the stagnant lymph being not as yet a solid tissue. The glands are so obscured by the overlying integuments that it is difficult to make out positively their exact condition, but those on the right side are certainly enlarged. Measurements of the legs give the following results :—

					Right.	Left.
Thigh at crutch ...	...	...	...	...	21½ inches	18½ inches
„ upper third	...	...	22	„	19	„
„ middle	...	...	...	20¾	„	17	„
Knee ...	...	...	...	...	18½	„	13½	„
Calf ...	...	...	...	...	15½	„	12½	„
Ankle ...	...	...	...	...	10½	„	8¾	„
Instep ...	...	...	...	...	10¼	„	9½	„
Base of toes	...	...	...	9¾	„	9½	„

One evening I examined his blood. One drop drawn at 6.30 p.m. contained one filaria; one drop drawn at seven p.m.

contained fourteen filariæ. It is evident from this persistence of embryos in the blood that the parent worms were not removed when the scrotum was amputated—at least, not all of them. From this fact, and the large number of embryos his blood contains, I believe there are several parent worms still in his lymphatics. The tumour he had on his left arm, which came and went so quickly, was, I have little doubt, caused by some obstruction of lymphatics brought about by filariæ.

7. *Cases of lymph-scrotum and elephantiasis of the leg combined.*

CASE XIX. *Elephantiasis of the leg; lymph-scrotum; varicose groin-glands; filariæ in lymph from groin-glands and scrotum, and also in the blood* (see Plate VI.).—TAIKOAN, aged twenty-eight; a farmer from Tchiupo, Baepi. No elephantiasis in his family, but in his village of 700 or 800 inhabitants he knows of four cases of elephantiasis of the leg, and four cases of elephantiasis of the scrotum. He drinks well-water of good quality, which, however, is stored in a jar, often for several days, and when the jar is refilled it is not always cleaned out. When thirteen years of age he had an attack of shivering and fever, with inflammation of the left leg and both groin-glands. He recovered in three or four days, but henceforward became liable to such attacks at very irregular intervals—sometimes only once or twice a year, sometimes as often as every month. With each attack the volume of the leg increased. The scrotum was similarly affected, and at the same time; occasionally it discharged, perhaps daily, perhaps once in three or four days. He never had chyluria. His body, generally, is in good condition. The right leg looks normal. The left leg is in a state of advanced elephantiasis, and a small ulcer has formed in front. Measurements are as follows:—

| Right calf | ... 12 inches | Left calf | ... 16 inches. |
| „ instep | ... 10½ „ | „ instep | ... 14 „ |

The left foot is very much expanded in all directions, and its skin is thickened, glabrous, and in thick folds at the flexures.

I

The groin-glands on the left side are much enlarged, are soft, varicose, and very prominent. Those on the right are similarly affected, but to a smaller extent, though still quite distinctly.

The scrotum is an excellent specimen of a lymph-scrotum; the contained lymph being sanguineous gives the parts a purplish tinge. A vesicle opened on the lower part emits, with considerable force, a stream of bloody lymph, and one can collect two or three ounces in as many minutes.

August 14th, 1879.—At 6.30 this morning I aspirated the left groin-glands and got abundance of bloody lymph in which active filariæ abounded. A quantity of this lymph, and also lymph from the scrotum, were put aside. At five p.m. the coagulum had contracted to one-third the bulk of the entire lymph; it was bright red, and floated in a straw-coloured fluid. In coagulum from the glands, on tearing off a piece and compressing it firmly between two strong slides, I saw many filariæ imprisoned in the fibrine, which restrained their movements, thereby making their detection rather difficult. No filariæ found in the serum of either gland or scrotal lymph. Next morning, twenty-four hours after the lymph was drawn off, the coagula in both specimens had disappeared, and the coloured corpuscles, sinking as usual to the bottom of the glasses, formed a dark brown sediment. In this filariæ were found, but not many. Blood from the finger, drawn at eight o'clock the previous evening, contained eight filariæ to the drop.

August 15th.—Aspirated, at seven p.m., the same gland, and most carefully searched two large slides full of lymph; not one embryo found. Aspirated a gland on the right side, and examined most carefully one large slide; not one embryo. The lymph from both glands was of exactly the same character as that drawn previously. About four drachms of lymph from each side was stood aside to await resolution of the coagulum and subsidence. Two slides of blood from the finger carefully searched, but no filariæ found; however, when the blood was again examined at 9.30 p.m., fifteen filariæ were found in one slide.

August 16th.—Pierced another gland on the right side at

six a.m. Bloody lymph in great abundance with plenty of filariæ; one slide contained six, another three; one slide of finger blood contained one. At six p.m. the coagula of last night's lymph had disappeared, a dark-brown sediment and a milky fluid taking its place in both glasses. In a full, large slide of the sediment from the left side lymph I found four active filariæ, but in a similar slide of the right side lymph I could not find one. The lymph drawn this morning still coagulated; but August 17th, six a.m, I note the coagulum had disappeared, and in one drop of sediment twenty-three active filariæ were found.

CASE XX. *Lymph-scrotum ; varicose groin-glands ; ele-phantoid condition of the skin of left thigh; filariæ in lymph from glands, but none in the blood.*—BEK, aged twenty-eight; a farmer from Tchiupo. Lives in a village with about 1,000 inhabitants, amongst whom he knows of two cases of elephantiasis of the scrotum, and two (a man and a woman) of elephantiasis of the leg. The woman is his mother. A brother and two sisters are healthy; his father is dead, apparently of phthisis.

The disease for which he applied commenced eight or nine years ago with fever, and two red, painful, and inflamed streaks on the inner surface of the left thigh, a little above the knee, and passing up to the groin. He says that the pain preceded the shivering and fever. The swelling at first was trifling, but similar attacks recurring about twenty times a year the swelling became more marked, and about a year ago the scrotum became inflamed and involved in the disease. The scrotum has inflamed now altogether seven or eight times. He never had chyluria, nor, unless when the leg and scrotum inflamed, fever.

The integuments of the left thigh over its inner, anterior, and posterior surfaces are distinctly elephantiased from the knee to a point about two-thirds up the thigh. The rest of the limb appears to be quite normal; but in the situation mentioned, the skin is darker than that on the corresponding part of the other thigh. It is also coarser, and cannot, especially about the centre of the affected patch, be pinched up in a fine fold, but feels brawny and as if anatomically

I 2

continuous with the subcutaneous tissue. When one of his usual attacks of fever sets in this patch of skin becomes red and distinctly swollen.

The groin-glands, both inguinal and femoral, and on both sides, are much swollen and are distinctly varicose. The scrotum is a good specimen of lymph-scrotum, and does not require further description.

I introduced a subcutaneous syringe into one of the varicose inguinal glands on the right side, and easily obtained a supply of milky lymph. In this, during a short and hurried examination, I found one perfect and rather languid filaria embryo. A large slide of blood from the finger was examined at the same time, but no filariæ were found in it. On the following morning I again aspirated the same gland, and procured a darker, and more bloody lymph; lymph was also drawn from the left femoral and left inguinal glands; in all of these, specimens of filariæ were found. A slide of blood from the finger was examined at the same time, but, as on the previous day, it was devoid of embryos. The patient did not remain longer under observation.

It may be objected that the affection of the skin of the thigh in this case was not elephantiasis. If it was not this, it is certainly a wonderful coincidence that his mother, who lived in the same house with him, exposed to the same chances of filaria infection, should develope true elephantiasis of the leg.

8. *Elephantiasis of the leg with chyluria.*

I have only once met with this combination, but the circumstances of this case are so significant, that I request the readers' particular attention to the narrative.

Case XXI. *Elephantiasis of the leg; varicose groin-glands; lymphous discharge from leg; filariæ in groin-glands, but not in blood; subsequent development of chyluria.* (Plate VII.) Tcheng, aged nineteen; a paper gilder from Amoy. There is no elephantiasis in his family, nor, as far as he knows, in his neighbourhood. About ten years ago was attacked with shivering and fever, accompanied by swelling and pain in the right popliteal space. The fever and great pain continued for about a fortnight, and the swelling for a month or two longer. An abscess formed, burst, and healed; but ever since a clear, yellow, lymphous fluid has distilled from the skin over the site of the abscess, and from the back of the calf of the leg. He says he has many attacks of fever every year, accompanied by pain, but no particular swelling of the leg or of the groin-glands. He has never had chyluria. His body is fairly developed for his age, notwithstanding the fever. The groin-glands, both inguinal and femoral, are much enlarged—those on the left side most so—and distinctly varicose. Those on the right—the side affected with elephantiasis—are slightly varicose, but not so prominent as on the other side, though still very large; they are also much more dense and firm to the touch. On inserting the hypodermic needle into a varicose gland on the left groin, abundance of dark red fluid was withdrawn. The fluid coagulated rapidly; and the coagulum disappearing after six hours, a copious dark red sediment collected at the bottom of the glass. In this sediment I found great numbers of living and active filariæ. The bulk of the sediment was composed of corpuscles like those of blood.

The right leg is enlarged from the upper third of the thigh downwards. Though rougher than healthy skin, the skin is not so rough, except on the foot, as it is in long-standing elephantiasis; but it is dense, adherent to the subjacent tissues, and in every respect like the integument characteristic of that disease. From the ham to the lower third of the leg, the whole of the calf, and part of the sides and front of the leg are covered with a sort of weeping eczema. Examined carefully the part of the skin thus affected is seen to be defined at its margin and slightly elevated, reddish on the surface, and finely papillated. No breach of surface can be detected, but on pressing firmly with the point of the finger a clear, yellow lymph is made to well up from the surrounding tissue, as if from a sponge. There are two firm elevations in the popli-

teal region about the size of pigeons' eggs, rough and encrusted
on the surface, badly defined at the base, and yielding much
discharge. These elevations represent the seat of the abscess.
Unlike ordinary elephantiasis the calf of the leg is the least
swollen part; and it is just this part that the discharge issues
from so copiously. Measurements of the legs:—

	Right.	Left.
Upper thigh	19 inches	16 inches
Middle „	18½ „	16 „
Knee	18 „	13 „
Middle calf	14½ „	12 „
Heel	16 „	13 „
Instep	12½ „	9½ „
Toes...	10 „	8 „

Three large slides of blood from a finger drawn at seven p.m.
contained no filariæ. Next morning at six o'clock two more
slides were carefully searched, but with the same result. The
leg was dressed with zinc ointment, and I note a week afterwards that the discharge had considerably decreased, the leg
feeling heavier and more stiff. Blood drawn from the finger
at seven a.m. was again examined, but was devoid of filariæ.

Three days later I note:—" There is now little discharge
from the leg. The right inguinal and femoral glands, with
the exception of the most internal of the inguinal glands,
feel more solidified. The latter gland is distinctly varicose.

" The following are now the measurements of the leg :—

Upper thigh	19 inches.	...	Heel	16 inches.
Mid thigh	18¾ „	...	Instep	12 „
Knee ...	19 „	...	Toes	9¾ „
Mid calf ...	14½ „			

"Left inguinal and femoral glands very prominent and
distinctly varicose. At 7.30 p.m. subcutaneous syringe introduced into left inguinal glands, and sanguineous lymph
readily obtained. About half an ounce was collected in a
glass and left to stand. Before coagulation two large slides
of this were examined, but no filariæ were found. The syringe
was again employed to abstract lymph from the varicose
gland already described as the innermost of the enlarged

glands on the right side; in one slide of this two languid filariæ were found.

"The glasses containing the specimens of lymph from both sides were now placed under cover to await resolution of the coagula, and the subsidence of any embryos they might contain. Twelve hours afterwards the coagula had contracted to one-sixth their original bulk; they had become of a bright red colour, and floated in a milky serum. In the sediment of the fluid and in the coagulum from the left side, several live embryos were found during a brief examination. The examination of that from the right side was very brief and imperfect, and discovered nothing. Next day, however, the coagula in both glasses had completely disappeared, and in the sediments of both many dead filariæ were found. Blood from the man's finger drawn at 9.30 a.m. (?) contained no filariæ."

A fortnight later I note :—" Withdrew by the canula of a hypodermic syringe about six ounces of a slightly sanguinolent lymph from the left inguinal glands, and also about two ounces of a similar fluid from the right inguinal glands. These, on coagulation and subsidence, after twenty-four hours, yielded a very few filariæ in the sediments. Blood from the finger, drawn at ten p.m., yielded no filariæ."

The last of these notes was made on August 19th, 1879; the patient then ceased to attend, and I lost sight of him for two years. On August 3rd, 1881, he turned up again with his leg and groin-glands pretty much in the same condition as they were two years before. But it was not on account of them he applied; he came to ask if anything could be done for a chyluria which appeared about a month before. His urine is constantly loaded with sanguineous-looking lymph. It was collected every three hours for a day or two, and was always more or less chylous; but, although the sediment was carefully examined, no filaria was found in it.

August 5th, six a.m.—About two ounces of salmon-coloured lymph was removed by hypodermic syringe from the enormously distended left inguinal glands; the sediment from this, after resolution of the coagulum, was carefully searched, many slides of it, but for a long time no filaria was discovered; at last three dead specimens were found. Blood from the finger was examined on—

August 4th, six p.m. and seven p.m., many times;

August 5th, 1.30 p.m., four p.m., six p.m., 6.30 p.m., 7.30 p.m., nine p.m., and midnight;

August 6th, six a.m.,

but not a single filaria was found.

On August 19th, I have a note that the sediment of six ounces of chylous urine was examined, but no trace of parasite was found in it.

These cases are part of the clinical evidence on which my belief in the parasitic causation of tropical elephantiasis is founded. The theory has been subjected to some amount of loose criticism, but no attempt of a serious or important character has been made, as far as I know, to explain away the interpretation I put on the facts I have recorded. Something has been said about coincidence, but surely the frequent combination of lymph-scrotum and elephantiasis is not in every case coincidence; nor is it fair to say that the supervention of chyluria in the case last narrated is simply coincidence. By such argument it would be possible to explain away every theory in pathology. Much has been made, too, of the absence of filariæ in the blood in fully-developed elephantiasis. But I have narrated several cases of lymph-scrotum in which they were absent in that fluid, yet were found in the lymph. It is nearly impossible to get gland-lymph in elephantiasis; were it otherwise we might find filariæ, or the remains of them, in it. Besides, we know that the parasite, after working much mischief, dies in some cases. May there not be something in the conditions of lymph circulation, or obstruction, in ordinary cases of elephantiasis, inimical to the life of the parasite which produced them, or that renders it impossible for its embryos to gain admission to the general circulation? An evanescent cause often, in pathology, produces a permanent effect. The gravid womb by pressure causes varicosity of the veins of the legs which does not disappear after parturition. Constipation in the same way causes hæmorrhoids; rheumatic inflammation of the valves of the heart permanent heart-disease, and so on. In the same way in elephantiasis, the parasite, after permanently damaging the lymphatics, disappears.

If we do not accept the parasitic theory as explaining tropical elephantiasis, then we are obliged to conclude that in the tropics there are two forms of this disease; that they affect the same parts of the body; are found in the same districts; are characterized by the same sort of fever, inflammation of the lymphatics, and skin-lesions; that in fact they are in every respect identical, and only differ in their ætiology. I think this is so unlikely that few on reflection will maintain it.

CHAPTER VI.

THE clinical evidence for the theory that the elephantoid diseases are caused by embolism of the
lymphatics by the ova of the filaria arranges itself
under two heads.

1. Cases to show that a frequent habitat of the
parent parasite is the lymphatic trunks on the distal
side of glands.

2. Cases in which the ova of the parasite were
found in lymph from the distal side of the glands.

1. *Cases to show that a frequent habitat of the
parent parasite is the lymphatic trunks on the distal
side of glands.*

I have already referred to the "finds" of the
parent worm by Bancroft and Lewis. In these
instances, the worm was certainly found on the distal
side of glands. I have also given several cases in
which the young of the parasite were found in gland-
lymph and yet were absent from the blood, giving
presumptive evidence that the parent must also have
lain on the distal side of the glands. The two follow-

ing cases prove that she, sometimes, at all events, lies there. The first case is the one referred to at page 1.

CASE XXII. *Lymph-scrotum; filaria embryos in lymph from scrotum, but not in blood; excision of part of the scrotum; parent filaria in dilated lymphatic.*—PHÆ, aged forty-six ; a pedlar and farmer from Phoolamkio, Iu Khæ.   Four or five years ago he noticed that after much walking had pain in both groins and along the course of the spermatic cords, but he says it was never, or very seldom, associated with fever. He has never had inflammation or abscess of the scrotum. At first there was swelling of, and pain in, the groin-lymphatics ; but on the bursting of a vesicle which had formed on the scrotum, and the discharge of much fluid, these subsided. During the first year or two scrotal discharges occurred only once or twice ; then, they became more frequent, and during the last three months the discharge has been nearly constant.   It may stop for a day or two occasionally, but, as a rule, the scrotum drips lymph night and day, perhaps to the extent of ten to fifteen ounces in the twenty-four hours.   The discharge, he says, is always clear like water, and when collected in a bowl, coagulum, with red particles and streaks on it, forms rapidly. He has never had chyluria nor any serious illness.

October 11th, 1880.—Inguino-femoral glands on both sides enlarged, especially on the right side ; they are neither distinctly varicose nor firmly indurated, but have a soft, spongy feel. The bulk of the scrotum is only slightly increased, but everywhere on its dusky-red surface are scattered innumerable minute vesicles, varying in size from a No. 6 to a No. 2 shot. Pricking any of these permits the escape of a clear watery lymph. As I examine the scrotum this fluid, oozing from some ruptured vesicles, drips constantly. The right testicle is absent, probably undescended ; there is no hydrocele on the other, which feels large and healthy. The under surface of the sheath of the penis is somewhat swollen, but is not vesiculated. The scrotum is soft and silky. There is no elephantiasis or swelling of the legs.

The clear watery character of the lymph is peculiar. I found in a short examination of sediment of some drawn at eleven a.m. to-day one embryo filaria. I collected two other specimens of lymph, one drawn between four and five p.m., the other at seven p.m., and stood the three lots to await resolution of coagula. Blood drawn from the finger at 7.45 p.m. had no filariæ; again, at eight p.m., examined a large slide, but found no filariæ. The blood is very watery and deficient in corpuscles.

October 12th.—Examined the sediment of the three specimens of lymph and found embryo filariæ in all of them, two or three in every slide of sediment. It is evident from this that the filariæ observe no periodicity while they are in the lymph, and that reproduction is a continuous process.

In this case I believe the obstruction in the lymphatic circulation is very low down, probably not higher than the inguino-femoral glands, and that it is complete; because, 1st, had the lymph regurgitated after passing through glands it would probably be milky, or sanguineous, and much richer in corpuscles than it is; 2nd, it is clear and watery, as it is near the radicles of the lymphatics; 3rd, there is an absence of marked varicosity of the lymphatic glands it first reaches—were the obstruction higher up the lymph circulation those lower glands would be distended by accumulating lymph; 4th, filariæ in the lymph, but not in the blood—proving that the obstruction is complete. I think it probable, considering these facts, that the parent worm is between the surface of the scrotum and the first lymphatic glands, and that we will find it when the scrotum is excised.

October 15th.—Removed part of the scrotum this forenoon. The dripping of lymph continuing I thought it advisable to operate to save this man's life. As he lay on the operating table under chloroform I could see the anterior border of the spleen bulging out the relaxed and wasted abdominal muscles, and could feel that the organ was very much enlarged. Under such circumstances I generally abstain from all serious operations, but when I recollected the corpuscleless and watery state of the blood, the absence of a history of malarial fever – the usual cause of splenic tumour here—the probability that it was the result of the state of the blood, and that this again was caused by the constant day and night dripping of lymph from the scrotum, I determined to proceed. The operation was a very simple affair. I dragged down the affected portion of the scrotum till it was clear of the testicle, transfixed the fold thus formed with a finger-knife, cut upwards and then downwards, removing a circle about two and a half or three inches in diameter of soft, spongy, watery scrotum. Only three arteries required ligature. Pressure with the palm of the hand over the right inguino-femoral glands forced from a varicose lymphatic in the upper and right corner of the wound a stream of lymph the thickness of a fine knitting needle, and with a projection of three or four inches. The lymph thus expressed was clear and watery. I failed to do the same on the left side. The solitary testicle—the left—was healthy. The edges of the wound were brought together and united with catgut sutures.

The scrotum, when excised, had been placed in a clean bowl, and when the operation was finished I took it up and carefully examined the cut surface. Finding nothing unusual I folded it up, intending to examine it at my leisure. However, being curious about my prognostication, I took it up again and unfolding and exposing the cut surface, saw wriggling on it very vigorously a long and slender worm, of a cat-gut, opaline look, the thickness of a medium-sized horse-hair. One end of the worm was free, the other entered the cut end of the lymphatic corresponding to that from which I expressed the lymph on the right side. About two inches of the worm was free. I tried to coax out the rest with my finger, but failed. The worm appeared to be working back again into the scrotum. Fearing it would succeed in this I laid it on the handle of a scalpel. When it had partly dried and adhered, I made gentle traction; but the worm snapping in the vessel, I procured only about two inches of the free extremity, with long pieces of uterine tubes and alimentary canal dangling from the transverse fracture of the integument. I did not attempt any further examination of the scrotum (which contains the caudal end of the female, and probably the male worm), but placed it in spirits and sent it to England. Dr. Bennett, of H.M.S. *Swinger*, was present at the operation, and saw the worm.

The same evening I examined with the microscope that part of the worm I had broken off. It was the head end of a female. The body was quite plain, without markings, and tapered rather abruptly to the simple, somewhat club-shaped mouth. The vagina opened about $\frac{1}{25}$-in. from the mouth; the uterus was packed with embryos at every stage of development. In the lower part of the uterine tubes the embryos lay at full length, outstretched as we see them in the blood; the sheath was very distinct in one of the embryos that had escaped from the vagina. The worm was certainly viviparous. The following are my measurements, carefully made:—

Greatest diameter of body	$\frac{1}{165}$-in.
Diameter of alimentary canal	$\frac{1}{900}$-in.
„ head at shoulder	$\frac{1}{450}$-in.
Orifice of vagina from mouth	$\frac{1}{25}$-in.
Diameter of body at vagina	$\frac{1}{125}$-in.
Ova before differentiation of embryo, cleavage complete ...	$\frac{1}{850}$-in. $\times \frac{1}{850}$-in.
Ova after differentiation of embryo $\frac{1}{590}$-in. $\times \frac{1}{700}$-in.	
Diameter of uterine tubes	$\frac{1}{800}$-in.
Free embryo	$\frac{1}{95}$-in. $\times \frac{1}{3000}$-in.
Length of sheath visible beyond the head of the free embryo	$\frac{1}{1400}$-in.

The animal was mounted in urine (of a specific gravity similar to that of lymph) for examination and measurement. In such a medium the parts retain their natural proportions; if mounted in water, glycerine, or spirits there is often much distortion, and an incorrect idea of relative and actual size produced.

October 15th.—Doing well. A slide of blood drawn at 5.30 p.m. from the finger contained no filariæ.

October 16th.—One slide of blood drawn at 5.30 a.m. contained no filariæ.

October 26th.—Had an attack of fever yesterday, and he is still hot. The sheath of the penis is considerably swollen, but otherwise the case is doing well; the wound is granulating kindly, and there has been no escape of lymph since the operation.

November 3rd.—Wound nearly healed; swelling of penis subsided. Patient, who has been taking large quantities of iron, much stronger; blood still very deficient in corpuscles; spleen smaller; one slide of blood drawn at six p.m. contained no filariæ.

November 6th.—Wound healed; no filariæ in the blood; going home to-morrow.

CASE XXIII. *Abscess in the thigh caused by the death of the parent filaria; varicose groin-glands; fragments of mature worm in the contents of abscess.*

January 7th, 1881.—A middle-aged, well-nourished man came to hospital to-day with a large, hard, brawny-red swelling in the upper and inner part of the right thigh. An abscess was evidently forming. I observed that the corresponding femoral glands are somewhat enlarged, softish, and not inflamed; and he said they had been swollen long before the present trouble began. He also had had fever, apparently lymphatic. Accordingly, I concluded that the glands were filarious, and that their enlargement was not secondary to the inflammation then existing. I drew off from them with a hypodermic syringe some milky lymph. In this a very imperfect and hurried search was made for embryos, but none were found. *Diagnosis.*—Abscess caused by death of parent filaria in lymphatics. Pus, apparently, had not formed, so mercurial ointment was ordered to be rubbed into the swelling, and poultices to be applied.

January 10th.—Returned this morning in great pain; matter had formed. Free incision gave vent to about four ounces of dark yellow-brown pus, in which floated two or three dark clots of blood, evidently effused for some time. The pus and clots were all collected, and this evening I carefully searched them. By drawing a needle rapidly through the pus I succeeded in entangling three or four fibres, which, on being subjected to microscopical examination, proved to be fragments of a mature female filaria. In one fragment were large numbers of fully-formed outstretched embryos, all dead and granular, great bunches of them escaping from rents in the wall of the uterus; other fragments were crowded with ova at an earlier stage of development (see illustration).

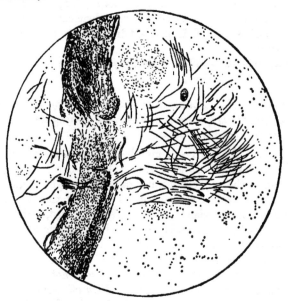

FRAGMENT OF FEMALE FILARIA SANGUINIS HOMINIS FROM ABSCESS IN THIGH, SHOWING REMAINS OF ALIMENTARY CANAL, DECOMPOSING BODY, DEAD EMBRYOS ESCAPED FROM RUPTURED UTERUS; ONE OVUM VISIBLE.

January 25th.—Filariæ have been found in this man's blood every night till date. To-night I found two active specimens in a slide of finger-blood drawn at seven p.m. The wound is healing, and the surrounding induration has disappeared; but the glands, especially the femoral, are still swollen on the right side. He tells me that these glands have been big—but on this side only—for over ten years, and that once, long ago, they were inflamed. For a year or two he has had very little fever, but formerly was more subject to it.

January 28th.—This afternoon pierced the enlarged femoral glands and drew off, rapidly dropping, about two ounces of salmon-coloured lymph. (Dr. Jamieson of Shanghai was present.) In one slide of this lymph found a very languid and faintly granular embryo. One slide of blood, drawn and examined at six p.m., contained one active embryo.

February 14th. — Two drachms of lymph drawn from glands. A full slide of this contained twelve active filariæ. One of these, examined with a high power, looked perfectly healthy and normal.

This man remained under observation for about two months after the abscess was opened, and therefore after the death of the parent filaria which was connected with the enlarged femoral glands; yet, during all this time, his blood contained at the usual hours a fair stock of embryos—apparently as many at the end of the two months as at the beginning. It is fair to infer from this, either that there were other mature female worms alive in his lymphatics; or, if the dead specimen removed from his thigh was the only one, that the young filariæ keep alive for several months both in lymph and blood.

These two cases are of themselves conclusive proof that a habitat of the parent filaria is the lymphatic trunks on the distal side of glands. The two following cases corroborate this statement likewise, for they prove that the ova of the worm have been found in these lymphatics; and, the ova having been found there, it necessarily follows that the parents that gave birth to them must have been in the distal lymphatics.

2. *Cases in which the ova of the parasite were found in lymph from the distal side of glands.*

K

CASE XXIV. *Filariæ in blood; enlarged, indurated, and partly varicose groin-glands; elephanto-œdematous legs; ova of filaria in lymph from groin-glands.*—OH, aged forty-four; a farmer from Tchangtchiu, Toana-sia. No elephantiasis in his family. There are about 1,000 inhabitants in his village. Years ago, he recollects, there was a man with a big elephantiasis scroti, who was killed by the Taiping rebels. The little boy who brought the patient to hospital has a huge elephant leg. Besides these he knows of no other cases of elephantiasis in his village. He generally drinks well-water, but when working in the fields often drinks from the paddy-field runnels. The well-water is stored in a jar, without a cover; the jar is filled every second day, but cleaned only once every five or six days.

He says he has had enlarged glands since boyhood, but never had pain or inflammation in them, nor have they altered in appearance much during many years. When very young—about twenty—had quartan ague for a month or two, but until last year had, on the whole, excellent health. Last year, however, in the fourth month, after indulging in a little wine, he fell asleep, and when he woke up had rigors followed by fever, but not so severe as to prevent him working. He noticed that his legs, both of them, had swollen. They remained enlarged for eight months, and on the inner side of the left thigh a pustular-like eruption broke out. By the beginning of the present year eruption and swelling had quite subsided, and he was in his ordinary state of health. In the fourth month he had a severe attack of fever and diarrhœa, during which the legs swelled again and acquired their present appearance. In the morning they are less, in the evening larger.

When he presented himself at the hospital he was excessively anæmic, but the swelling of the legs was too brawny for the ordinary œdema of anæmia, yet too soft for the hypertrophy of elephantiasis. It readily pitted on firm pressure. The heart and urine were normal. The inguinal and femoral glands on both sides are much enlarged, and in shape characteristic of *filaria sanguinis hominis;* but they are firmer and more solidified

than those generally met with in lymph-scrotum, and softer
than those usually associated with elephantiasis. One gland
in the left groin — the uppermost and outermost — felt
slightly softer than the others, and a hypodermic syringe
drew off from it a small quantity of perfectly clear lymph.
In this lymph I found eleven ova, presumably of *filaria
sanguinis hominis*, and one languid free embryo. The ova
were all advanced to the last stage of development; each
contained a perfect embryo, which moved about inside the
delicate wall in a rotatory fashion, just as I had seen the
embryos of *filaria immitis* of the dog, when they had
descended close to the vaginal end of the uterus. The ova
were oval, the extremities of the long diameter having a
tendency to "point." Their dimensions were $\frac{1}{500}$-in. ×
$\frac{1}{750}$-in. I saw no trace of lash in the embryo. In one
slide of blood from the finger, taken at the time the lymph
was abstracted from the gland (early in the morning), four
filariæ were found. Two days afterwards I pierced the
same gland and abstracted a small quantity of bloody
lymph. In this I found neither ova nor embryos; but
following the needle, as it was withdrawn, there escaped a
drop or two of bloody lymph, and in this I found thirty-five
active and free embryos, but no ova. At the time of this
last examination blood from the finger contained twelve
embryos to the drop. A similar examination, made two
days later, yielded one embryo in the lymph, but no ova.

CASE **XXV.** *Lymph-scrotum; filariæ in lymph from
scrotum, also ova containing coiled-up and active embryos; small
number of parasites in the blood: operation.*—TUI, male, aged
fifty; Tchangtchiu, Khiotau; a farmer. There are some 200
to 300 inhabitants in his village, including several cases of
elephantiasis. One, called BENGA, I operated on some years
ago, removing a 12-lb. scrotum.

When young was careless about the water he drank, taking
it indiscriminately from pool, well, or river. When a little
over ten years of age had frequent attacks of ague, both
quotidian and tertian. His scrotal trouble began at eighteen.
He had hydrocele then, and at times inflammation of the

scrotum and lymphous discharges. Two years ago, he says,
I tapped his hydrocele. I forget the circumstance and the
character of the fluid withdrawn; as I did not inject iodine,
doubtless at the time I considered the hydrocele to be of
filarious origin, although he says the fluid removed was clear
and straw-coloured. The hydrocele did not return, but the
scrotum enlarged. He has attacks of fever and enlargement
of the groin-glands; and, irregularly, some three to ten times
a month, the scrotum discharges a clear fluid, very like urine
in appearance.

May 18th, 1881.—The scrotum is as large as a pumelo, and
the penis is buried in it; the upper and anterior part is firm,
like a forming elephantiasis, while the lower and back part is
covered with enormously dilated lymphatics, some of the
ampullæ, containing clear fluid, being as large as the tip of a
finger.

Seven p.m.—Pricked a vesicle; profuse discharge of fluid, in
which I found filariæ. A slide of blood from the finger, drawn
at nine p.m., contained no parasites.

May 19th, six a.m.—Slide of finger-blood examined; no
filariæ. Lymph drawn last night again examined; it had
coagulated but feebly; it again yielded filariæ. The feeble
coagulum was now broken up by stirring. It rapidly disappeared, a small quantity of red deposit and some white
cloudy flocculi subsiding. In this sediment were many
embryos; and, in nearly every slide, ova with active embryos
struggling vigorously to stretch their chorional envelopes.
No double outline could be detected in the embryos. The
chorion could be distinctly made out, especially when the
activity of movement had somewhat subsided.

May 20th.—An assistant examined a large slide of blood,
drawn at ten p.m. last night, and in it found one embryo; and,
again, at six a.m. to-day, but then found none. I examined
several slides of sediment from the lymph of the 18th, and
found embryos still alive, many of them enclosed in an oval
or nearly globular sac, and two specimens in which the
chorion was half stretched. These latter embryos were still
working vigorously, but had not quite completed the stretching operation, as a third of either anterior or posterior end

was still doubled on the rest of the body, no room having as yet been gained for the animal to lie completely outstretched.

In this man a very few embryos still found their way into the circulation, but there certainly was no free communication between the lymphatics of the scrotum and the blood.

May 21st.—Scrotum removed, skin of penis being preserved. I quite expected to find the parent worm in this case, but although the scrotum was cut up into very small pieces and carefully searched no trace of the animal was observed. The tissues were much more dense than is usual in lymph-scrotum, and their bulk was considerably greater than obtains in the generality of these cases. In fact it appeared, but for the vesicles and discharge, more like an ordinary case of elephantiasis. No lymph could be made to regurgitate by pressure on the groin-glands.

June 10th.—Case doing well. Since the operation the blood was frequently examined, and at suitable times, but no filariæ were found in it.

CHAPTER VII.

DISTOMA RINGERI AND ENDEMIC HÆMOPTYSIS.[*]
(Plates VIII., IX.)

THE list of parasites inhabiting the human body is gradually becoming a long one ; another addition—the latest, I believe—has been recently made by Dr. Ringer, of Tamsui, Formosa.

The following notes embrace all that is yet known of the new parasite.

Some time ago, November 6th to December 18th, 1878, I had in hospital here (Amoy) a Portuguese suffering from symptoms of thoracic tumour, presumed to be an aneurism. He improved with rest and treatment, and returned · to Tamsui whence he had come, and where he had resided for many years. He did not live long after his return. He died suddenly (June, 1879) from rupture of an aneurism of the ascending aorta into the pericardium. Dr. Ringer made the post-mortem examination, and, knowing I took an interest in the case, kindly wrote me the particulars of the examination. Besides describing the immediate cause of

[*] Reprinted from "Customs Medical Reports," No. 20, p. 10.

death, he told me he had found a parasite of some sort in making a section of the lung, and promised to send the animal to me for inspection.   He wrote:—

" After making a section I found the parasite lying on the lung-tissue—it might have escaped from a bronchus.   Whilst alive a number of young (microscopic) escaped from an opening in the body   There were some small deposits of tubercle, no cavities, and, if I remember aright, slight congestion of the lungs."

Last April a Chinaman consulted me about an eczematous eruption he had on his face and legs. The eruption had been out for some time, and had its origin, he believed, in an attack of scabies. Whilst he was speaking to me, I observed that his voice was rough and loud, and that he frequently hawked up and expectorated small quantities of a reddish sputum.   At that time I was making examinations of lung-blood in connection with another subject, and as this man's sputum afforded a favourable opportunity for examination I placed a specimen under the microscope.   The sputa, which to the naked eye appeared to be made up of small pellets of rusty pneumonic-like spit, specks of bright red blood and ordinary bronchial mucus, contained besides ordinary blood and mucus corpuscles, large numbers of bodies evidently the ova of some parasite.   These bodies were oval in form, one end of the oval being cut off and shut in by an operculum, granular on the surface,   blood-stained,   measuring   on   an   average $\frac{1}{800}$-in. × $\frac{1}{500}$-in.   Firm pressure on the covering glass caused them to rupture and their contents to escape, the shell being left empty and fractured at

the opercular end. Though empty the shell had a
pale brownish-red colour. No distinctly organized
embryo could be made out in the uninjured ovum,
but when the contents were expressed they resolved
themselves into oil masses, and granular matter
having very active molecular movements. A delicate
double outline could be made out in most of the ova.
They were so numerous that many fields of the microscope showed three or four of them at once.

Two days afterwards I again examined this man's
sputum, and found it full of ova as on the previous
occasion. I asked him to come again, and to supply
me from time to time with sputum, but he did not
return, and has left the neighbourhood, I believe. I
hoped to attempt successfully the hatching of the ova,
as has already been done in the case of other disto-
mata; but his disappearance, and my failure to get
another and similar case, oblige me to postpone the
experiment.

At his first visit I obtained the following particulars of his case:—

Case XXVI.—Tso Tong, male, aged thirty-five; native of
Foochow; a secretary in the salt office; resident in Amoy
about one year. He was born in Foochow city, and lived there
till he was twenty-one years of age; he then went to Tecktcham, a town in North Formosa, about two days' journey from
Tamsui, and resided there for four years; then he returned
to Foochow for a year and a half. He was again sent to
Tecktcham for a second service of four years. He returned
again to his native town for a year, and was then sent for
six months to Henghwa. Afterwards he lived successively
in Foochow, one year; Amoy, a year and a half; Foochow,
four months; and again Amoy for one year, where he is at
present stationed. A year after his first arrival in Tecktcham,
when he was twenty-two years of age, he first spat blood.

Every day for nineteen days he brought up from half an ounce to an ounce of blood ; he emaciated slightly, but had very little cough. Hæmoptysis returned about six months later, smaller in quantity, but, as in the former attack, the blood at first was pure, unmixed with mucus, and of a bright red colour ; this second attack lasted for a few days only. Since then he has spat blood for two or three days at a time in small quantities every second or third month. He has never had much cough, and he says that the blood is always mixed with mucus after the first mouthful. Once, during two years, he had no blood-spitting. Though rather thin he enjoys good health. I could discover no signs of lung-disease on auscultation. His father is dead, but not from cough; his mother, who died ten years ago, had a cough. He has had two brothers and two sisters ; they are all of them alive and in good health.

When I discovered the ova in this man's sputum I recollected Dr. Ringer's parasite, and that the Portuguese in whose lung it was found had also for many years lived in North Formosa ; and I came to the conclusion that this Chinaman's lungs probably contained a similar parasite, and that it was the cause of the blood-spitting. At my request Dr. Ringer sent me the solitary specimen he had found a year before. It was preserved in spirits of wine. I placed a little of the sediment in the spirit under the microscope, and found in it several ova of the same shape, colour, and dimensions as those I some time before found in the Chinaman's sputum. Most of the ova were ruptured ; a few, however, were still perfect. The parent parasite was spatula-shaped, of a light-brown colour, firm leathery texture, and measured $\frac{14}{32}$-in. $\times$ $\frac{5}{32}$-in. $\times$ $\frac{1}{32}$-in. It was evidently a distoma ; but not feeling quite sure if it was a new species or not, I sent it to Dr. Cobbold. He pronounced it to be new, and has named it *distoma Ringeri*, after the discoverer. Referring to the specimen, he says:—

"I satisfied myself that the fluke was new to science, and accordingly I propose to call it *distoma Ringeri*, after the discoverer. Though mutilated, the oral sucker was well shown, as also were traces of an organ which I regarded as the remains of the ventral acetabulum. When flattened on a glass slide, the capsules of the vitellarium were well seen, and occupied fully four-fifths of the body, lying deep under the dermal surface. The worm reminds me very much of *distoma compactum*, which many years ago I detected in the lungs of an Indian ichneumon, but it is much larger and evidently a distinct species." ("Journal of the Quekett Microscopical Club," No. 44, August, 1880).

We are as yet not in a position to say much about the pathological significance of this parasite. I do not think it common in this locality, but when practising in South Formosa I recollect seeing many cases of chronic and oft-recurring blood-spitting without apparent heart or lung lesion, and it is just possible that the hæmoptysis in many of these cases was caused by *distoma Ringeri*. My patient told me blood-spitting was a very common complaint in Tecktcham.

The intermediary host or hosts, the geographical distribution, and the mode of entrance of the parasite into the lungs offer a very interesting field for future investigation.

DISTOMA RINGERI AND ENDEMIC HÆMOPTYSIS—
*continued.**

In the "Customs Medical Reports," vol. xx., page

* Reprinted from "Customs Medical Reports," No. 22.

10, I called attention to a new parasite, the mature form of which had recently been discovered by Dr. Ringer in Tamsui, Formosa. I therein succeeded in associating this animal with a peculiar form of recurring hæmoptysis, common in one part at least of the Chinese Empire, which had hitherto not been understood; and I gave some particulars of a case occurring in my own practice, in which the association was apparent. At that time I was unaware that Professor Baelz, of Tokio, had been working at the same subject, and it was not until I read, in the "Lancet" of October 2nd, 1880, a summary of a paper by this gentleman, that I learned that this disease had been described by him, and that it was not uncommon in Japan. Although Professor Baelz, in the paper I refer to, errs in calling the bodies which I have proved to be the ova of *distoma Ringeri*, gregarinæ, yet, though I do not know the dates of his investigations, the merit of priority in the discovery probably rests with him.

In my report I mention that in making a post-mortem examination of a Portuguese dead of aneurism of the aorta, Dr. Ringer found a parasite in the lungs; that in the sputum of a Chinaman suffering from a chronic intermitting hæmoptysis I found certain bodies I had no difficulty in recognizing as the ova of a parasite; and that when these bodies and the ova emitted by *distoma Ringeri* were compared, they were found to be identical in size, shape, colour and contents.

Of the parasite discovered by Professor Baelz, the "Lancet" says that it is

"Met with in two forms: (1) as yellowish-brown ovoid

bodies of ·13 mm. long and ·07 mm. wide. They have a double contour, from a translucent wall, ·02 mm. thick, which in different positions appears greenish or reddish, and at the larger end is a kind of cover, at which the cyst opens. The contents consist of delicate jelly-like material, in which are imbedded three or five aggregations of smaller bodies. The latter consist (a) of spherules about twice the size of a white blood-corpuscle, colourless, with sharp outlines. Around these spherules, and more or less enclosing them, is (b) a coarsely granular material scattered through the jelly, and in it molecular movements may often be seen. When the spherules have left the cyst, they show for a time the same movements, and then become invested with the granular substance, and become motionless."

These bodies, he concluded, are a stage in the development of gregarinæ, and he therefore proposes to call the disease they are connected with *gregarinosis pulmonum*, and the parasite *gregarina pulmonum* or *gregarina fusca*.

As the above description applied pretty accurately to the ova of *distoma Ringeri*, and as they were associated with hæmoptysis, I concluded they were identical, and wrote to Professor Baelz, requesting him to send me a specimen of the characteristic sputum from Japan. He very kindly did so, and I had no difficulty in seeing that the bodies he described were identical with those I was familiar with, and with the ova of *distoma Ringeri*. Indeed, in his letter to me, the professor says that both he and Leuckhart had already suspected they might be the ova of a distom. That this view is the correct one will receive additional and corroborative evidence in the sequel.

During the last eighteen months I have made many unsuccessful attempts to find the ova of the parasite in the sputa of natives of this district. I suppose I have examined altogether about 150 individuals. Therefore, it is not at all likely that the disease is common in Amoy and its neighbourhood. It is quite otherwise, however, in North Formosa, though only separated from us by some 200 miles of sea. Being anxious to attempt the development of the embryo, and despairing of finding supplies of ova in Amoy, I applied to my friend Mr. John Graham, of Tamsui, to find me some sputa. He answered my letter by sending me two bottles full of ova-laden sputum, one of which was filled by his house-boy, the other by his coolie. Dr. Johansen also recently sent me six specimens of sputum, three of which contained ova in abundance; of the ova-laden sputa one came from his hospital assistant, the other two from peasants living near Capsulan, a place about forty miles to the southwest of Tamsui. The facility with which these cases were found proves that the parasite must be very common about Tamsui; and Mr. Graham's servants, who some time ago both visited Amoy, told me that hæmoptysis, such as they themselves suffered from, was extremely common. Regarding their acquaintances, one of them said that 20 or 30 per cent., the other that 15 per cent., spat blood. Possibly these are over-statements, but at all events they show that the disease is extremely prevalent. With regard to Central and South Formosa, I recollect very distinctly my surprise at the large number of cases of hæmoptysis I used to meet with there, and have now little doubt that in *distoma Ringeri* we have the explanation.

The geographical distribution of this parasite is peculiar, if it is the case, as seems probable, that it is

rare or entirely absent on the mainland of China.
We have Professor Baelz's authority for its existence
throughout Japan. I suspect, therefore, that there is
something in the soil or geological structure common
to Japan and Formosa, but not present on the neighbouring continent, that determines this apparent
caprice in the distoma area; and that this geological
element, whatever it may be, is one necessary to the
existence of the intermediary host. The distribution
of similar parasites depends principally on the distribution of their intermediary hosts; this fact can
easily be understood. Both Japan and Formosa
resemble each other in being volcanic, and are both
members of that long string of volcanic islands that,
stretching along the eastern coast of Asia, includes,
besides these, the Loochoos, the Bashees, the Philip-
pines, and a host of smaller islands. I believe that
extended inquiry will show that *distoma Ringeri*
exists in all of these.

Endemic hæmoptysis can readily be diagnosed.
There is a history of irregular intermitting hæmoptysis associated with a slight cough, and, in the intervals of more active bleeding, the expectoration once
or several times a day of small pellets of viscid, brownish mucus. Violent exercise is apt to produce profuse hæmorrhage, and irritation of the lung, in any
way so as to induce coughing, causes the discharge
either of quantities of blood or of the characteristic
sputum. At the same time there are no objective
symptoms of lung-disease, and the patient probably
enjoys good general health. Examination of a small
portion of the sputum with the microscope at once
settles the diagnosis. I many times examined sputa

from the two cases I had under close observation for a considerable time, and never failed to find abundance of ova, sometimes counting as many as 20 in a single field.

The following are short notes of the two cases I refer to. I am told they are typical examples of the disease as found in Formosa.

CASE XXVII.—HENG, male, aged thirty-one; resides in Sinhang, Tamsui, where he works as a house coolie. His family, he says, is quite healthy; his mother, aged forty-four, and three brothers and four sisters are alive and well. His father died at fifty-eight of dropsy, and a sister died in childhood of small-pox. He himself is liable to ague. He was born in the town of Banka, and lived there till his eighteenth year; then he lived in Kelung for two or three years; afterwards he removed to Hobe, Tamsui, where his home has been for the last ten years. He has travelled about the north part of the island a good deal; been in Tektcham two or three years ago; and eight years ago accompanied some Japanese to Khilai, on the east coast, where he resided for upwards of a month. His blood-spitting dates from eleven years ago; he was then working on the tea hills, with his father, near Banka. At first he noticed, when he breathed hard in carrying heavy burdens, that he coughed a little and brought up mucus mixed with blood; from that time till now has spat blood more or less constantly; some days none, other days a considerable quantity. Once when pulling in a boat about two years ago he suddenly brought up over a bowlful of pure blood; but, as a rule, unless exerting himself violently, he only brings up a few drops mixed with the mucus. Sometimes he does not spit for a few days, perhaps a month on end, and then the hæmoptysis recurs, to last for one or two months. He has a slight cough, but on auscultation nothing much amiss can be detected. His thorax is very finely developed. He says that he never exercised discretion about the water he drank, especially when young; used to take it from river, well, paddy-field, or ditch, whichever lay most convenient, and he says that nearly all North Formosans are similarly indiscreet.

HENG lived in my house from the 14th to the 31st July, and during the whole of this time he could nearly always cough up blood or ova-laden mucus such as I have described.

CASE XXVIII.—HEÔ, male, aged twenty-two; born and resident in Hobe, Tamsui; a house-boy. Father and mother are both dead, both of them of some dropsical affection. Until he was eighteen years of age, enjoyed excellent health; then, without any obvious cause, he began to spit blood, especially after making any very great exertion. During one year, many times each month, he continued to spit blood, about an ounce at a time. He then got lighter work and the bleeding ceased, and has not recurred; but he has a cough still, and almost every day expectorates pellets of tenacious, muddy, yellowish-brown mucus. Sometimes for several days, if the weather is fine and his work is light, there is no cough or spit; but when the weather changes, or he has to exert himself, the cough and spit return. He complains of some pain about the left nipple, but the lungs appear healthy. His sputum is as described, and abundance of ova can be found in it.

When examined with the microscope, the ova of *distoma Ringeri* are seen to be shaped very much after the fashion of a fowl's egg, with the exception that a circular operculum about half the breadth of the egg closes the broad end. On an average they measure about $\frac{1}{300}$-in. $\times$ $\frac{1}{500}$-in., but some specimens are slightly larger and others slightly smaller. There is considerable diversity likewise in shape, some being more globular than the majority, whilst others are more elongated and tapered towards the narrow end. Their colour, which, when blood is entirely absent, as is sometimes the case, imparts the characteristic brownish tinge to the sputum, is a dirty reddish brown, and appears to reside both in the shell and in the granular portion of its contents. The shell is without markings, and shows in double outline more especially when it has been fractured by pressure. When viewed with a high power the ovum is seen to contain one, two, or more well-defined, pale sarcode globules embedded in a structureless matrix containing abundance of irregularly disposed dark granular matter. Usually one of these sarcode globules is brighter and better defined than the rest. By careful focussing they are seen to be made up of very minute granules in a state of active molecular movement. Pressure ruptures the shell at the opercular end, forcing out the contents, which resolve themselves into innumerable globules of all sizes, from fine microscopic granules to large bodies $\frac{1}{3000}$-in. in diameter. The smaller particles exhibit very active molecular movements, and tend after a time to coalesce round the larger. No trace of a differentiated embryo can be distinguished. . Once or twice I have seen attempts at yelk cleavage, a dozen or more elongated cell-like bodies with a bright nucleus in each occupying the whole of the interior of the egg; but never anything more advanced than this.

It is evident, therefore, that some time must elapse before an embryo can be sufficiently developed to start on the independent existence which has been found to be the first step in development in those distoms whose early life history has been studied. Reflecting that the ova are deposited in the sputum, that this affords probably their only

L

means of escape from the human lungs, and that they are placed in it with a purpose, I concluded that by following out the destinies of a sputum I should probably be set on the right track for working out the first stage at least of the history of *distoma Ringeri*.

When sputum is cast on the ground one of three things may happen: first, it may be eaten by earth-worms, molluscs, or other creatures; second, it may dry up and mix with the soil, the solid parts of it being, perhaps, afterwards blown about as dust; third, it may be washed and carried away by rain into well, ditch, pond, or river. I considered that if in any of these ways the ova are borne to suitable incubating media, the last is the most likely to favour the development of the distoma, and most in consonance with what happens in the case of better-known species. Accordingly, I determined to imitate nature as far as I could in this direction, on the supposition that rain or water was the first agency that operated on the ova.

I procured two supplies of sputum from the man HENG; one lot I placed, without admixture of any sort, in a wineglass, and covered it up, keeping it for comparison and future experiment; the other lot, measuring about one ounce, and containing many thousands of ova, I shook up with about an equal quantity of filtered well-water until the mucus, blood, and ova were thoroughly diffused. This was divided into about equal portions between six wineglasses, and water sufficient to fill the glass was added to each. These were numbered 1, 2, 3, 4, 5, 6, and placed under a glass shade in a room where, during the subsequent steps of the experiment, the thermo-

meter ranged between 80° and 94° F. Next day
No. 1 was not disturbed, but all water, except the
drachm or two at the bottom of each glass, containing
the sediment and ova, was removed by means of a
syringe from 2, 3, 4, 5, and 6, and fresh water added.
On the following day 1 and 2 were not disturbed, but
3, 4, 5, and 6 were again watered, and so on. Thus
in No. 1 the ova were washed once, in No. 2 twice, in
No. 3 thrice, in No. 4 four times, in No. 5 five
times, in No. 6 six times, the washings taking place
at intervals of twenty-four hours.

My notes of observations show that no development occurred in the unwashed ova ; that it was
delayed in No. 1, where only one washing had
been performed ; that it advanced steadily without much notable difference in 2, 3, 4, 5, 6,
until at the end of from six weeks to two months
the majority of the ova produced active ciliated
embryos. A small quantity of sediment from one
or more of the glasses was removed with a pipette
daily, or every second day, and examined under the
microscope. Ova were always easily found. For the
most part they were entangled in little flakes of
miscellaneous *débris*, but from this they could easily
be separated. Notes were made of the various
changes as far as they could be detected ; but for
the first few weeks, on account of the dark, granular
character of the contents, it is difficult to say precisely
what the different steps were that led up to the
formation of the mature embryo. Great molecular
activity can be detected in the paler globules for some
time ; then these lose their distinctness, large oil
globules appear about the periphery of the yelk, and

a paler mass shows in the centre. In time the latter contracts, leaving the shell by a considerable space. Languid movements ensue in it; these become more active; a ciliated epithelium is developed on its surface, and an indentation at the opercular end indicates the presence of a mouth of some sort.

On the twenty-sixth day of incubation I note :— Examined some sediment from No. 3, and in it found an ovum of characteristic shape and colour, with an embryo in it possessing considerable activity and plastic power. It moved vigorously in the shell, and altered from time to time the shape of its body, which, for the most part, was heart-shaped, a distinct depression existing at the opercular end. Contents of the body granular. No vessel visible. No cilia visible when in ovo, but on crushing the egg the ruptured embryo escapes and its collapsed integument is then seen to be covered by long cilia, which keep in active movement for about one minute. Examined No. 4, and found several ova with active embryos of the same character. Also No. 1, but in it there appeared to be no advance in development.

On the twenty-eighth day I note :—In all the glasses, except No. 1, the ova contained ciliated embryos. If carefully expressed, the embryo retains its activity for eight or ten minutes after its escape. It rushes off from the egg a globular, ciliated, rotating ball; as movement subsides the body elongates, and a ciliated epidermis is seen to extend from the tail as far forward as the anterior third or shoulder of the animal. The anterior part is naked, and at its apex is provided with a papilla or beak.

The body of the animal evidently lies free in the shell, the cilia motionless at this stage and directed backwards. If we watch the anterior part or head, which is always directed to the operculum, and for the most part closely applied to it, it is manifest that this is fixed in some way. By careful examination of ova at a later stage of development, I have satisfied myself that this is effected by an involution of the delicate membrane lining the shell, which here becomes continuous with the ciliated epidermis of the body; thus the neck is surrounded by a sort of collar, which keeps it a fixed point. The movements of the animal, during the last few days of its residence in the egg, appear to be directed to rupturing this connection, for the head is first turned forcibly to one side, then to another, expanded, contracted, and jerked about, as if the little thing were annoyed and irritated by the collar restraining it. When this has been ruptured the embryo moves about in the shell, trying in an excited sort of way to escape, the cilia vibrating rapidly. Frequently, failing to force the operculum open, it turns completely round and energetically butts the opposite pole of the ovum with its head. After a time it succeeds in opening the operculum, which is either carried completely off, and may be found lying at some distance, or is thrown back as if on a hinge.

If we rupture an ovum very carefully a week or two after the appearance of the cilia, and are successful in extruding the little animal without crushing its delicate tissues, it will move away from the shell a short distance, its body elongating and contracting, and the cilia playing rapidly for a few minutes.

Gradually all movements will cease, the body passing from heart-shape to spade-shape, the handle of the spade being represented by a minute papilla with a very fine canal, apparently opening at its apex. Now it may be distinctly seen that the ciliated epidermis does not cover the fore part of the body, only the posterior two-thirds, extending as far forward as the rounding in of the shoulder ; also that the epidermis is in plates, one covering the tapered posterior end, and two other indistinct lines in advance of this indicating that altogether there are three or four such plates or bands. Soon after extrusion the homogeneous or finely-granular contents present larger globules containing actively moving granules, and as the feeble contractions of the body and ciliary motions cease, these granular globules increase in number, until finally the entire mass is made up of minute dancing micrococcus-like particles. Then the epidermic plates roll up, leaving the body quite naked, the cilia fade from view, and finally an amorphous mass is all that remains.

If, however, we rupture the ovum at a later stage of development, or if our observations are made just when the embryo has squeezed its plastic body through the natural opening, the behaviour of the embryo is somewhat different. First, the cilia are seen to start into rapid motion, and then, after a preliminary pause, to rupture and separate itself from the lining membrane of the shell which is sometimes forced out entire along with it, or, apparently to consider what has happened, the animal rushes off at great speed, gyrating about after the manner of certain infusoria. From time to time it pauses, contracting itself into a

perfect disc or globe, rotating rapidly on its axis, first
in one direction, then in another.   Anon, it dashes off
to a distant part of the slide, exhibiting in its course
many diversities of form.   When going at high speed
the body is much elongated ; at a less speed oval, or
fiddle-shaped, or square ; but at no time is the beak
or naked shoulder protruded as long as the animal is
alive and active, a slight depression on the ciliated
surface alone indicating where these are retracted.
Beneath the epidermis is a thick contractile layer ;
the interior appears to be fluid or a soft jelly, holding
minute granules in suspension, and sometimes a larger
bright point can be detected.   No vessel of any sort
can be traced.   I do not know how long the animal
preserves this active ciliated form.   I have kept one
alive in a glass cell for over twenty-four hours (Plates
VIII., IX.),

Such, briefly, is the history of the first step in the
development of *distoma Ringeri.*   The ova are laid
into the bronchial mucus; in the sputum they are
cast on the ground ; by rain, or other means, they are
carried to stagnant water; they sink to the bottom ;
in the course of six weeks or two months ciliated
embryos are developed ; when mature these force
their opercula, and swim free in the water.   What the
next stage may be can only be conjectured.   Doubtless, they enter the body of some fresh-water animal
to undergo further metamorphoses.   Perhaps this
animal is eaten by man, or, possibly, the parasites once
more obtain their freedom, and, while still in the
water, are swallowed, and thus obtain an opportunity
of gaining access to the human lungs, their final
destiny.

I have not spoken yet of the fate of the unwashed
ova. The glass containing them was not disturbed
for about three weeks. At the end of this time the
sputum had decomposed, stank abominably, and had
settled into two layers; one upper, more or less clear,
and a lower, turbid and dark brown. On sampling
the lower layer, into which the ova might be supposed
to have gravitated, but few specimens could be found.
These, however, were, as far as I could judge, in no
way different from perfectly fresh specimens. The
sputum was then washed repeatedly with fresh water.
But, although in the sediment ova were numerous, no
decided advance in development could be detected; on
the contrary, in many, signs of decomposition were
apparent at the end of two months. In others, again,
the characteristic globules of sarcode could still be
distinguished. Thus it would appear that unless the
ova are freed from mucus and have access to fresh
water within a short time of their birth, they perish.
If, however, water is supplied to them soon after they
leave the lungs, though in limited amount, as was
done in the case of glass No. 1, they do not rot, but
retain their vitality, proceeding slowly in development. In the case of the ova in this glass the embryos were not differentiated till about the fortieth day.

It is evident, therefore, that the ova must be brought
into contact with water, and that this is the medium
through which the parasite, and the disease it produces,
pass from one human lung to another. In the history
of this parasite we have another argument, if such is
needed at the present day, for a pure water supply.
Not many months ago there were few who would not
have laughed at the idea that blood-spitting could be

produced by a draught of dirty water. Now this
connection can be demonstrated. How many more
diseases acknowledge impure water as one of the
most important factors in their etiology, time and the
advance of science will show. This matter of *distoma Ringeri* and endemic hæmoptysis may have
little practical interest for any but some 40,000,000
or 50,000,000 of Asiatics and the few hundreds of
Europeans who live among them, but it is a valuable
text for the advanced sanitarians of Europe to work
on and preach from ; to show, that to-morrow some
new fact may disclose unsuspected connections between
disease and uncleanliness.

By these observations the search for the intermediary host is limited to a comparatively small group
of animals.   It must be an inhabitant of fresh water ;
it is common to Japan and Formosa ; it does not in-
habit or is rare on the mainland of China,—at least
that part of it near Amoy.   The latter circumstance
has precluded me from pursuing the investigation
further, but I trust it will be taken up and successfully completed by some one residing in Formosa or
Japan, who, being in the midst of the disease, must
enjoy ample opportunity.   The limitation of the field
in which investigation need be made must simplify
the search ; but that it will be a short and easy one
does not follow.   The history of the liver fluke, the
cause of so much disease in sheep, is not yet complete, notwithstanding the great inducements and
facilities offered to its investigators in Europe and
elsewhere.*

* Since this was written, the beautiful researches of
Thomas on the metamorphosis of the liver fluke in *Limnæus*

On discovering the cause of endemic hæmoptysis, the first thought that suggests itself is the possibility of curing it. Could the parasite be killed, the disease would be arrested. An important point bearing on this question has yet to be ascertained, and that is the exact site of the parasite in the lungs. Is it free in the bronchi, or is it jammed into the branches of the pulmonary artery? If the former, the parasite may be dislodged; if the latter, the prospect of cure must be very small indeed. An autopsy is necessary to settle this point, and I trust our *confrères* in Japan will bear this point in mind when they get the opportunity. The exact position of the mature parasite could easily be ascertained by microscopical examination of bronchial mucus; the appearance of ova in a particular tube would show that the animal is to be found by following up that lead.*

Proceeding on the assumption that the parasite had its habitat in the bronchi, I made several attempts in the two cases I have given to kill or dislodge it. I caused the patients to inhale the spray of solutions of various drugs atomized by a Lister's steam apparatus. In this way the tincture and infusion of quassia, the infusion of kousso, solutions of turpentine and santonine in spirits of wine were introduced into the lungs. In addition to these the man HENG inhaled

truncatulus have been published, and an important blank in the life-history of a destructive parasite filled in (see "The Quarterly Journal of Microscopical Science," January, 1833).

* For some very valuable observations by Dr. Cobbold on the lung flukes, see the reports in the medical journals of a discussion on the subject at the meeting of the Medical Society, March, 1883.

the vapour of burning sulphur. Inhalation was practised twice daily for a week in one instance, and for a fortnight in the other. . Certainly before these men passed from under my personal observation they were improved so far as cough and expectoration were concerned, but in both instances a small amount of ova-laden sputum could still be procured by irritating the lungs and inducing cough; they returned to Tamsui before I could be sure that the cure was complete. In reply to my inquiries, Mr. Graham wrote me lately that HENG still spits small quantities of blood at long intervals, but that HEO has now no cough and can no longer bring up distoma mucus. He, possibly, is cured.*

I am sorry I have not been able to carry further these experiments in treatment. I would not allude to them now had I much prospect of being able to extend them. I mention them only in the hope that others, with opportunities better than those I enjoy, will pursue the inquiry in this very practical direction.

Our knowledge of the history of the ovum, and the medium in which it is developed, indicates the direction which effort at prevention should take. But

* I had an opportunity of examining HEO three months after the attempts at cure above described. He said he was quite well, that he had lost his cough, had spat neither blood nor mucus, and that he regarded himself as cured. I caused him to inhale irritating substances, and thus forced him to cough violently, but he failed to bring up any trace of distoma sputum. He told me that my other patient, HENG, still spat blood; and he also brought me three specimens of ova-laden sputum from three of his friends in Tamsui.

I fear our knowledge in this instance is a little in advance of any practice we may look for in a Formosan. Europeans who happen to be stationed in Formosa, or who may be travelling in the island, will understand from these remarks the necessity for extra caution with regard to drinking water. They should never neglect to boil or filter it when the least suspicion is entertained about its purity. A little neglect in this matter may be paid for with a chronic hæmoptysis.

CHAPTER VIII.

WHILE making a post-mortem examination of a
Chinaman on September 21st, 1881, I encountered in
the abdomen a number of animals belonging to an
order of parasites which have not hitherto been
found infesting the human subject, although common
enough in certain of the lower animals. The specimens I brought to England and submitted them to
Dr. Cobbold, who has pronounced the species to be
new to science, and has named it *ligula Mansoni.*
I cannot say if this parasite has any pathological
importance. I mention the matter here in the hope
that attention having been directed to it, other
observers, with better opportunities for post-mortem
examinations in Orientals than I enjoy, may be
induced to look for this new parasite and work the
matter out.

In the post-mortem referred to the parasites were
found in the loose areolar tissue behind the kidneys,
and in the subperitoneal areolar tissue in the flanks
and iliac fossæ. One specimen was found free in the
right pleural cavity. They were twelve in number.
Some were coiled up in a loose knot, others again
were slightly extended. They could be seen through

the peritoneum, and when this was incised were easily dragged out of the loose subperitoneal fascia. In colour they were dead white, and when extended at full length measured twelve to fourteen inches in length, by one-eighth of an inch in breadth, and one-sixtieth in thickness; the two extremities were rounded off and rather thicker than the rest of the body. To the naked eye there were no transverse or other markings visible, although the general appearance of the animal, its shape, colour, and languid vermicular-like movements forcibly reminded one of a tapeworm. Unfortunately, I had little leisure at the time for a careful microscopic examination, but this much I made out, that one extremity was lipped, and the other had a short longitudinal slit in it. The whole of the body was occupied by a vast number of clear spherical bodies, each having a double or treble outline and distinct nucleus; these were held together by a loose fibrous matrix and very thin transversely striated integument. Slight pressure caused the matrix and integument to split up longitudinally and rupture transversely. I made out no trace of alimentary or generative organs.

Specimens of these parasites were shown at the Linnæan Society, and at the same time a very interesting paper on the subject of "Ligulosis" was read by Dr. Cobbold.

The following are my notes of the case and post-mortem examination in which the parasites were found. The case is further of interest as illustrating some of the points I have already discussed when treating of *filaria sanguinis hominis*.

CASE XXIX. *Lymph-scrotum and elephantiasis scroti com-*

*bined; profuse discharge of lymph; great debility; filariæ in
blood and lymph; operation; death; post-mortem examination;
ligula Mansoni in abdomen.*—TCHHAI, aged thirty-four; a
cotton carder from Tchin Kang, Tchhiah thoh. No particular
family disease; no elephantiasis in his village.

He stated that his scrotal trouble began, when he was twenty-
six years of age, with an attack of fever and inflammation
ending in abscess. After the first attack fever and inflammation of the scrotum frequently recurred. Six years ago
scrotal discharges appeared for the first time; then the scrotum
was much larger than at present and very tense. About ten
months ago he had a long series of regular ague attacks, first
quotidian, then tertian, and finally quartan in character;
altogether he was ill with this fever for seven months. He
suffered from cough and anorexia. Latterly, for about a
month, the discharge from the scrotum has been nearly constant, running him down to a state of excessive debility.

September 2nd, 1881.—The scrotum is larger than a man's
head, and the penis is buried in it. Of the groin-glands the
femoral, especially those on the left side, are most affected;
they are large and varicose. Only one or two on the right
side are involved. The greater part of the scrotal tumour
feels and looks like an ordinary elephantiasis, but on the
right, and more especially on the left side of the mass, there
are groups of large tense vesicles—the group on the left side
occupying an area the size of the palm of the hand. Also,
on the upper part of the tumour, about two inches from the
orifice of the prepuce, there is a long dilated lymphatic about
an eighth of an inch in diameter. Lymph is constantly escaping in a fine stream from a vesicle on the right side of the
scrotum, and from any vesicle that is handled at all roughly.
Several pounds of lymph must have escaped to-day. It is
white, like watery milk, coagulates, and contains filariæ.
Several were found in a short examination of lymph drawn
at eleven a.m. to-day. Blood drawn at 6.30 p.m. contains
filariæ. There is no elephantiasis of the legs, nor is there any
history of chyluria.

September 3rd.—Although the man was in very bad health,
and in addition to his other troubles had symptoms of stric-

ture of the œsophagus,* his only chance appeared to be from
an operation on his scrotum. The profuse and uninterrupted
lymphorrhagia would certainly kill him in a very few days.
I accordingly removed the scrotum to-day. It weighed over
three pounds, and exhibited the usual structure of a lympho-
elephantoid tumour. A hernia on the right side, firmly
adherent to the bottom of the scrotum, had to be dealt with,
and gave some trouble in dissecting up. Dilated lymphatics
in the upper and outer angles of the wound discharged lymph
profusely and had to be ligatured.

September 21st.—The case did well for some time after
operation. There was no recurrence of the lymphorrhagia,
but the difficulty of swallowing from the strictured œsophagus
increased, and made the administration of a sufficiency of
nourishment impossible. Dysentery then set in and he died
this morning. At the time of his death, the wound, though
indolent, was quite clean, and in no way responsible for the
fatal termination.

Post-mortem Examination.—Body very thin; feet œdematous. Abdomen—bladder too full; whole of the large intestine covered with ulcerations from ileo-cœcal valve to anus;
no adhesions or signs of peritonitis; two lumbrici in the
stomach, and about a dozen in the small intestine; the parasites I have already described under the peritoneum. Thorax
—normal except the œsophagus; this, where the left bronchus
passes over it, was thickened and adherent to the bronchus;
the lumen of the tube was so constricted that it could not be
traversed by the little finger, and on slitting it up a thickening and ulceration occupied a complete segment of the tube
for about an inch and a half at the situation indicated; I could
not pronounce the thickening to be cancerous; the ulceration
on the mucous surface was very ragged and irregular, and
one little hole extended through to the interior of the left
bronchus. In the left bronchus were two full-grown lumbrici,

---

* Stricture of the œsophagus is a remarkably common
disease in Amoy. I have never been able to satisfy myself
as to the cause of this frequency. I do not think that the
strictures are malignant or traumatic.

which doubtless had crept up from the stomach after death and found their way to the lungs through the ulceration in the œsophagus. The lymphatics of the groin over the saphenous opening, especially the left, were firm, but not hard. They gave the idea that the outer part of the gland had at one time been distended, but had collapsed enclosing a firm nucleus. The lumbar glands were also enlarged. I examined blood from the lungs and found in it a few filariæ; also blood from the spleen, and this too contained a few filariæ; lymph expressed from the left groin-glands contained filariæ in considerable abundance.

I regret I was unable to make a more minute examination of the lymphatics.

CHAPTER IX.

TINEA IMBRICATA, AN UNDESCRIBED SPECIES OF BODY RINGWORM.*

DERMATOLOGISTS pretty well agree in their descriptions of the various forms of epiphytic skin disease, and in the characters of the vegetable parasites with which they are associated. Favus, tinea tonsurans, tinea decalvans, chloasma, are distinct diseases, and are generally recognized as such. This unanimity, however, does not obtain in the case of *tinea circinata*, or ringworm of the body, some authorities teaching that there are several species of tinea included under this name, while others affirm that there is but one disease, and one species of fungus producing the different modifications. Dr. Tilbury Fox is one of the most recent writers advocating this latter view. In his work on skin diseases he is very decided in his assertions. He says, referring to this subject, "It will be seen that I include a number of diseases hitherto regarded as distinct from *tinea circinata* under that head. Of the correctness of this step I have no shadow of doubt, and it really saves a vast addition to the vocabulary of the dermatologist."

* Reprinted from the "Customs Medical Reports," No. 14.

Under one head he brings, besides the typical form of *tinea circinata*, all what he calls its uncommon phases, "such as general parasitic tinea, parasitic eczema, Burmese ringworm, eczema marginatum, Malabar itch, Chinese itch, etc.," and these varieties of the disease he attributes to the influence of diversity of climate, clothing, constitution, and part of the body affected.

While agreeing with Dr. Tilbury Fox in the desirability of simplifying so complicated a subject, with all deference to his high authority I take the liberty of asserting that his generalization is too sweeping, and that there are at least two distinct and well-marked species of body ringworm. I agree with him thus far in considering that the names he enumerates do not *always*, or generally, represent different species of disease; but when he maintains that there is only one species, he goes too far, and, I believe, is mistaken. It seems strange that one so practised in observation should fall into this error. I can only account for it by supposing that he and those whose opinions he represents have never seen a case of the disease I propose to describe under the name of *tinea imbricata*, and that a careful description of its characteristics is not to be found in medical literature. In the following remarks I will endeavour, by a detailed account of a case of *tinea imbricata* and another of *tinea circinata*, to supply this description, and bring out the characteristics of the two diseases by their contrast; and, afterwards, I hope to show by a description of the microscopic appearances of their respective fungi, and the results of experiments in inoculation, that the difference is not only in clinical

M 2

characters brought about by peculiarities of circumstance, but actually in species, and is everywhere and in all circumstances constantly maintained.

Details of a Case of Tinea Imbricata and of a Case of Tinea Circinata.

CASE I. *Tinea Imbricata.*—LIAM, male, aged forty-five; a rice grinder; native of, and resident in, Amoy. He is well nourished, muscular, and in excellent general health. Twenty years ago he emigrated to the Straits Settlements, where he worked in a sago factory, but returned to Amoy after an absence of only three years. He came back in consequence of the eruption of the skin disease he now suffers from, his friends having told him it would disappear in the cooler and drier climate of China. He was in the Straits but a few weeks when the inner surface of his right thigh was attacked by the disease, which, in the course of three years and a half, spread over nearly the whole of his body. At the sago factory there was a Cantonese who had the disease. This man's towel he used to wipe his body with, and to this circumstance he attributes his infection. There has been no remission all these twenty years; his skin has all along had the same appearance. During the winter, perhaps, the itching which troubles him so much in warm, damp weather, is mitigated.

The extent of the disease is most easily described by enumerating the parts not involved. These are: 1. A symmetrical patch of sound skin, extending in front from over trochanter major to trochanter major; on an average this patch is about four inches broad; in the middle of the body it expands slightly and includes the genitals. 2. An oval patch in the middle line over the lower lumbar vertebræ; it is about the shape and size of the palm of the hand, its long diameter lying vertically. 3. A symmetrical patch in front of the chest, including both nipples and stretching from armpit to armpit, the skin of the walls of which, both brachial and thoracic, is quite healthy. This patch measures over the sternum about six inches in breadth. 4. The whole of the hairy scalp, with the exception of that over the occiput, the disease on which is continuous with that of the neck. These four patches of sound skin are shaped and arranged symmetrically; but, 5, a long irregular surface on the front of the left leg has nothing corresponding to it on the right side. With the exception of the parts enumerated the whole of the rest of the skin is implicated.

It would be difficult to give a description applicable to the disease as it is seen in all parts of the body, but if I select one spot some idea of what I might call the plan of the disease may be conveyed.

The patch selected is situated just above the right nipple. On the surface of this the epidermis is arranged in a series of wavy lines, lying parallel to each other, and having a more or less concentric arrangement in relation to an imaginary point situated somewhere about the tip of the right shoulder. It is very like the ringed appearance in a cross-cut log of wood. On closer examination, this effect is found to be produced by an undermining of the epidermis, giving rise to long flakes, about one-eighth of an inch in breadth, the free edge of the scale being directed towards the centre of the circle, the convexity remaining still firmly attached. If the hand is passed over the surface from the circumference towards the centre of the circles, the scales are smoothed down; if in the reverse direction, they are raised up, and stand out prominently, defining the wavy outline of the rings very distinctly. If we attempt to detach the scale it is found to be firmly adherent at the outer edge; but by using a little force it can be peeled off, the flake becoming thinner, softer, and more delicate the further we proceed from its original attachment, until it is completely separated. If the forceps is carefully used, two or more inches in length of epidermis can thus in some places be separated in a continuous, unbroken ribbon. Just under the free edge of the scale, the skin is lighter in colour than between it and the preceding or succeeding rings. The rings are about one-eighth to one-quarter of an inch apart, so that thirty can be counted between one corner of the square and the other. Some are quite regular in their outline over a

length of five or six inches; others, again, are interrupted at
intervals, and more or less irregularly convoluted; but there
is no spot an inch square within the area of the disease unoccupied by these scaly rings.

On the soft and protected skin of the thorax and abdomen
the disease and its characteristic features are seen in their
greatest perfection.   On the back and shoulders the flakes of
loosened epidermis, being seldom disturbed by scratching or
friction, have acquired greater dimensions, but from their
size and the irregular way in which they have been shed,
they more or less conceal the ringed pattern so evident in
front.   The arms and legs, feet, hands, and face being
subject to much friction have assumed a rough, reddish,
furfuraceous appearance, with the wavy outline of the rings
only visible in places.   The hair of the eyebrows and occiput
seems quite healthy, growing strong and glossy through the
diseased epidermis.   Though rough to the touch from the
desquamation, there seems to be no thickening or effusion
into the corium, notwithstanding the length of time the
parts have been affected.

In this case, as observed at present, the line of demarcation
between the perfectly sound and the diseased skin is not very
abruptly marked.   It looks as if the disease endeavoured at
times to push on to, and establish itself in, the sound skin,
but finding the ground unsuitable, released its hold, leaving
little outposts of spots and lines at intervals along the ground
it has been compelled to abandon.

Over the abdomen, the rings have advanced from right to
left, the free borders of the scales being directed to the right;
over the thorax on both sides, diagonally from above downwards and without inwards; over the back from a point
between the shoulder-blades.

Another point deserving of particular notice is the existence
of symmetrically arranged patches of leucoderma on which
there is no scaling or rings.   Such patches are to be seen on
the anterior surfaces of the wrists and forearms; and still
more markedly on the upper, anterior, and inner surfaces of
the thighs.   The disease has been in existence longest in these
localities.   In the leucodermic patches the loss of colour,

though extending over a considerable area, is not in one large continuous patch; but white spots, an inch or more in diameter, are mixed with spots of the natural colour of the skin, giving the places mentioned a piebald appearance.

During all the years this man has lived in Amoy, he is not aware of having communicated his disease to any one.

CASE II. *Tinea Circinata.*—TCHOK, male, aged nineteen; came to hospital suffering from general debility and ring-worm.

The characters of *tinea circinata* are well known. A minute description of them is therefore unnecessary. In giving this case I will merely mention the principal and diagnostic features, to insure its being recognized as the disease in question.

On his face, and nowhere else, is a well-marked ringworm. It has been out for one month only, and spread from a spot on the right side of the nose. The ring is incomplete on the right cheek, and is broken in several other places, once by the right eye, again by the mouth, and again by the left *ala nasi*. On an average, it is about a quarter of an inch in breadth; it is slightly but distinctly elevated, of a dark red colour, scurfy and obscurely vesiculated at places, and is very itchy. The margin is more abrupt at the spreading, shading off at the receding edge; and though there is a tendency at the convex border to undermining of the epidermis, the scales so produced are very minute, not in any place measuring more than $\frac{1}{4}$-in. × $\frac{1}{32}$-in. There is no attempt whatever at reproduction of a ring in the skin already travelled over, which is quite natural in colour and texture. Under the microscope mycelium and spores of trichophyton are to be detected in scrapings from the ring.

Trichophyton Tonsurans and the Fungus of Tinea Imbricata.

The microscopic appearances of the fungus of *tinea imbricata*, although in many respects closely resembling those of the fungus of *tinea circinata* (trichophyton tonsurans), are yet sufficiently distinctive to render the diagnosis of the disease by the microscope alone quite a simple affair. In the first place, it is often no easy matter to find fungus elements in *tinea circinata*, and several slides may have to be examined before a fragment of mycelium, not to mention a chain of conidia, is found. But in the case of *tinea imbricata*, one has only to raise any scale on the diseased surface, and place it under the microscope, to see fungus elements in enormous abundance. In every field are hundreds of conidia, arranged in chains, crossing and re-crossing each other, and mixed with a fair proportion of mycelia; and with a little alteration of the focus one can see that there is not one, but several layers of this elaborate network. This contrast in the quantity of fungus in any given specimen is most remarkable.

Another point of contrast is in the position the fungus occupies in the skin. There can be no doubt about this in *tinea imbricata;* it is always in the lowest layers of the scale of epidermis. From the size of the scale, which can be raised and laid on the slide smoothly and accurately, this is easily determined. In the case of the fungus of *tinea circinata*, we cannot be so certain from microscopic evidence alone of its position; but the mycelial threads seem to spring from deep in the skin, and wind in and out amongst the superjacent layers of epidermis. The seat of *tinea imbricata* is undoubtedly in the non-vascular rete Malpighii, or deeper layers of the epidermis; of *tinea circinata*, probably in or on the surface of the vascular corium and its hair follicles; hence the small amount of irritation and inflammatory change excited by the former, and the thickening, induration, and red raised ring of the latter.

Additional proof that the rete Malpighii supplies the pabulum on which the fungus of *tinea imbricata* lives, is afforded by the absence of colour in the skin just travelled over by the rings of advancing disease, and by the frequent occurrence of leucodermic patches in those parts which have been longest affected, and the subsidence of the disease where the skin fails to reproduce its pigment layer.

Fungus of Tinea Imbricata (see Plate X.).

Conidia,—generally oval, rarely circular, often irregular, measuring from $\frac{1}{10000}$-in. to $\frac{1}{5000}$-in. in diameter, arranged in single rows, or long, often-branching chains. They appear to be formed in two ways, either by division of previously existing conidia, or by segmentation of mycelium. Where the latter has recently been effected, the conidia are more rectangular, of a darker colour, and often contain reddish-brown granules; otherwise the conidia are colourless, without markedly granular contents, and of a rounded contour. If a chain of conidia is traced to its termination, this is usually found to consist of a longer and larger spore, in some instances exhibiting a transverse constriction, as if dividing. In an ordinary specimen these chains of conidia are much more numerous than the accompanying mycelial threads.

Mycelium varies in breadth from a very minute thread up to $\frac{1}{5000}$-in. It appears to be of two sorts, a paler and a darker, though intermediate forms can usually be found also. The paler variety is less sharp in outline, and from its rounded appearance resembles more than does the other the structure of the perfect conidia ; it branches frequently, is interrupted irregularly by articulations and delicate transverse septa, and frequently terminates or arises in a chain of conidia.. The darker variety is more tape-like in its appearance, and is recognized by its delicate but sharply-defined border, and the numerous granules of dark, reddish-brown material it contains. This latter form is also frequently branched, and little protuberances are attached to it at intervals; it is much articulated in places, and terminates in a bulbous extremity or in a chain of conidia. The colour granules tend to run together when the specimen has been immersed some time in dilute liquor potassæ. Both forms of mycelium vary much in diameter, and the threads are but slightly bulged and only at long intervals.

Stroma.—This I have not recognized with certainty in recent preparations; but if the scales are kept for several weeks in a dry bottle, and then examined, it will be found that the conidia have nearly entirely disappeared, their place being taken by large, articulating, much-branched mycelial threads and patches of what I believe to be stroma. This latter is made up of innumerable exceedingly minute globular cells, heaped together without any definite arrangement.

As in all cases of epiphytic skin disease, bacteria, micrococci, and similar low forms of life abound in and about the epithelial scales.

Fungus of Tinea Circinata (Trichophyton Tonsurans).

Conidia.—In proportion to mycelium, and compared

to *tinea imbricata*, very few indeed, many scrapings having to be searched before they are found. In size they are much the same as those of *tinea imbricata*, but are more globular in form, and are often compressed in the direction of the axis of the short chain in which they are generally arranged. The terminal conidium is large and bulbous and more oval. They are generally seen to be connected with myeelium.

Mycelium varies in breadth, as does that of tinea imbricata, but it is distinguishable from the latter by numerous swellings and constrictions and other irregularities in outline. This contrast is very noticeable. It is frequently articulated to form conidia, and septa and branches are common. Generally the threads contain very minute dark granules. The course of a mycelial thread of *tinea imbricata* is usually long, straight, or gently curved; that of the mycelia of *tinea circinata* is generally short, irregular, and much convoluted.

Stroma, I have not detected with certainty.

Experiments in Inoculation.

The contrast in the clinical features of these two diseases, and the microscopic characters of their fungi, is decided. If I now show, by careful observation of the results of their successful inoculation, that these distinctive features are transmitted and maintained in every instance and in the same individual, the assumption of Dr. Tilbury Fox and others, that the disparity in the appearance of the varieties of ringworm is produced by differences in climate and other circumstances, will not hold.

Inoculation of Tinea Circinata.

I inoculated two assistants by scratching the epidermis on anterior surface of forearm, and rubbing into the spot scrapings from the ring of Tchok, Case 2. The inoculated spot was protected by a pledget of cotton wool held in place by strapping. The following are my notes, made every few days during the progress of the inoculation :—

5th day.—Dressings removed. One case has completely failed; but on the forearm of the other, close to, but not quite over, the seat of inoculation, is a very minute vesicle.

8th day.—A red, itching spot, slightly, if at all, elevated, about $\frac{3}{16}$-in. in diameter, where the vesicle was.

10th day.—Yesterday, the original inoculation spot became itchy and red, and to-day is larger and more itchy. The other spot, where the vesicle was, has not extended.

15th day.—The site of the inoculation is now occupied by a circular patch, $\frac{7}{16}$-in. in diameter. It is red, rough, slightly elevated, and itchy, and is beginning to assume the appearance of a ring, the centre being paler than the circumference and distinctly depressed. The site of the vesicle is now included by the ring.

17th day.—The ring, gradually enlarging, is now over $\frac{5}{8}$-in. in diameter, perfectly circular, abrupt towards sound skin, shading off towards centre, elevated, very itchy, with one or two minute vesicles on it. Trichophyton easily found in scrapings.

19th day.—Ring is now $\frac{3}{4}$-in. in diameter, $\frac{1}{8}$-in. in breadth, with a bright red, slightly furfuraceous surface; no large scales.

22nd day.—Ring is now $1\frac{3}{16}$-in. in diameter, rather more scurfy and less elevated; the minute furfuraceous scales are attached at the outer border of the ring; loose on the inner.

24th day.—Ring nearly $1\frac{3}{8}$-in. Skin in the centre appears to be quite healthy.

26th day.—Diameter about one inch. Outline more irregular.

28th day.—Ring is now oblong, irregular, and faded-looking; greatest diameter measures 1¼-in.

33rd day.—Ring measures 1¾-in., but is now not complete, being interrupted in several places. Outline also is more or less irregular in shape and colour. In places there are bright red spots, in other places paler spots; and some of these are in advance of the general body of the disease. Centre is quite healthy. The disease was to-day destroyed by the application of iodine liniment.

During the progress of the inoculation, the fungus was looked for from time to time, and always found. Its characters were those of trichophyton tonsurans, already described, and corresponded, as did all the other features of the inoculated disease, with those of the ringworm from which it was derived.

Inoculation of Tinea Imbricata.

I was anxious to make a successful inoculation of *tinea imbricata* in the same individual, and accordingly, as soon as I was convinced that the inoculation of *tinea circinata* had healed, I inoculated his other arm with scales from a case of *tinea imbricata*. These scales were quite two months old, having been kept in a stoppered bottle all the time. There was no result. I then sent for the man LIAM, Case 1, and, with fresh scales procured from him inoculated the left forearm in two places, front and back, treating the spots in exactly the same manner as I had done when on the same man I inoculated tinea circinata.

6th day.—Dressings removed. At the seat of inoculation the epidermis has been shed, leaving a very fair ring of undermined epithelium surrounding the spot, which is about ¼-in. in diameter; it is not elevated or altered in colour, though rather more glossy than the surrounding skin.

Fungus was searched for, but was not found. The shedding
of the epidermis I look upon as the result of the irritation, and
in no way the consequence of the fungus.

8th day.—Appearance much the same as two days ago,
though, possibly, more distinct. No trace of fungus in scales,
and no itching.

10th day.—The circle of desquamating delicate epithelium
has disappeared, but now there is a minute brownish spot on
each seat of inoculation, that on the back of the arm being
double. These spots are about $\frac{1}{16}$-in. in diameter, and do not
itch.

12th day.—The brown spot on the anterior surface of the
arm is slightly larger; it is not at all inflamed or very
distinctly elevated, and does not itch. The epidermis covering
it is very delicate, and a considerable flake of this is easily
peeled off by piercing it, and running a needle between it and
the corium. Transferred to the microscope, this is found to
be crowded with mycelium and innumerable chains of conidia
of the same character as found in the case of *tinea imbricata*
already described; the mycelium is perhaps more plentiful
and made up of shorter lengths, and in many of the threads
are large quantities of brown pigment-granules arranged as
nuclei. The spot on the back of the arm he has scratched;
it is red, denuded of epithelium, and crusted in consequence.

13th day.—The spot in front is now $\frac{1}{4}$-in. in diameter, of
a brownish colour, hardly elevated, and is surrounded by a
delicate overhanging fringe of detaching epidermis. That
on back of arm still damaged by the scratching; one half is
occupied by a small crust, the other half resembles the spot
on the front of the arm. It is red and swollen.

17th day.—The spot has now assumed a distinctly ringed
appearance, and measures $\frac{3}{8}$-in. in diameter. He says it itches
more than does the *tinea circinata* on the other arm, and has
in consequence been scratched and rather spoiled. In *tinea
circinata*, the surface of the ring is convex; in this it is ridged
like the crest of a breaking wave. I believe this degree of
elevation is, partly at least, attributable to the scratching. If
carefully analysed, the spot is found to be made up of a series
of concentric rings. From without, inwards, they are—1, a

brownish-red ring, about $\frac{1}{16}$-in. in breadth, lying apparently under the epidermis; 2, the red elevated ring, from the ridge of which a complete circle of delicate, detached epithelium springs, its free edge looking inwards; 3, a pale ring, with a glossy surface, surrounding 4, a central brown slightly raised spot, about $\frac{1}{8}$-in. in diameter. Ring on the back of the arm is not so distinct, and is not elevated. No redness or thickening of the skin; but there is a slight deepening of colour at the outer margin, a distinct ring of delicate scales, a paler circle, and a darker spot inside, just as on the front of the arm; diameter of spot $\frac{3}{4}$-in. Fungus in both plentiful.

18th day.—The spot in front is slightly larger, and a second ring of undermined and scaling epidermis is forming in the centre of the first; this second ring is $\frac{1}{16}$-in. in diameter. The brown central spot visible yesterday has disappeared, and the surface it occupied is now paler than normal. The patch on the back of the arm is also larger, but as yet there is no second ring forming, the central brown spot being still very distinct.

19th day.—Spot on anterior surface: Outer ring over $\frac{1}{2}$-in. in diameter, inner ring $\frac{1}{4}$-in. Spot on posterior surface: $\frac{9}{16}$-in. in diameter, without a central second ring, but the included space is frayed, and looks as if it had been well scratched. He says the itching is now much less troublesome.

24th day.—Ring in front nearly $\frac{3}{4}$-in. in diameter. A third ring is now forming. On the back of the arm the eruption is more irregular. A third spot on the same arm, the result of another and later inoculation, is proceeding typically.

27th day.—The patch in front is now $\frac{9}{16}$-in. in diameter, and a third ring has formed.

29th day.—A fourth ring has formed on both spots. No thickening or signs of inflammation. Scales are kept small by frequent washings. Ring in front nearly an inch in diameter.

31st day.—Four rings distinct and perfect.

36th day.—Five rings. There is now considerable irritation, especially about the outer rings, and a tendency to

inflame and vesiculate; the circles are in consequence not so
perfect. Greatest diameter nearly 1¼-in.

41st day.—The weather has become very hot, and probably
in consequence, the irritation in the spots has increased. The
inner rings have been spoiled by scratching, but the two outer
rings are quite distinct, though slightly inflamed. Diameter,
1⅜-in. The spot on front of arm protected by a cover, the other
spots destroyed with iodine liniment.

Several days afterwards, when the covering was removed,
the patch was found much inflamed; the rings could be traced,
but the fungus apparently had died, as the disease made no
further progress. The roughness and scaliness of the epidermis gradually subsided, and the part became natural in
texture, though from the slight alteration in the colouring of
the skin, the site of the rings could be traced for weeks
afterwards.

These experiments were repeated in two other cases with
similar results.

. From this description of a successful inoculation,
the nature and distinctive characters of *tinea imbricata*
can easily be made out. After inoculation, as in *tinea
circinata*, there is an incubation period of about nine
days. At the end of this time the fungus has multiplied sufficiently to slightly elevate the epidermis
under which it is growing, and form a brown mass
between it and the corium. When this has attained
a diameter of about ⅜-in., the epidermis in the
centre gives way; but, as it is still organically continuous with the sound skin at its margin, it is not
completely shed but remains a fringe round the
central hole. By friction or other means, the free
edge of the scale is from time to time removed; and
the brown central fungus and the tissues it is mixed
with, now no longer protected by a closely adhering
epidermis, are rubbed off as far as the attachment of

the scale, and the exposed corium appears pale. Just beyond this point the advancing fungus shows through the epidermis as a brown rim, perhaps very slightly elevated, about $\frac{1}{16}$-in. in breadth. When the entire ring thus formed has attained a diameter of about $\frac{1}{2}$-in., · a brown patch is again seen to be forming at its centre; this in its turn also cracks the young epidermis over it, and a second ring is formed inside the first, which it follows in its extension. A third brown central patch is formed in the centre of the second circle, and behaves in exactly the same manner; and so on with a fourth, fifth, and never-ending series of concentric rings.

There is a marked contrast between tinea circinata and. tinea imbricata in the parts and extent of the skin they respectively attack. The former elects, in preference to any other locality, those parts of the body which are usually covered with hair, as the scalp, axilla, and pubes; the latter, on the contrary, avoids these situations. The Chinese have very seldom a strong crop of hair on the front of. the chest, on the small of the back, or legs and arms; yet these situations, so frequently covered with hair in the European, are, strange to say, shunned by the fungus of *tinea imbricata.* If, however, *tinea imbricata* has spread on to a hairy part, the hair follicles are not invaded by the fungus, as in *tinea circinata,* and the hair continues firmly implanted, glossy, and natural.

Again *tinea imbricata,* if it has been in existence any length of time, involves a very large surface, as an entire limb, or side of the trunk, or oftener still, if not checked, nearly the whole surface of the body. *Tinea circinata,* though sometimes including in its rings large areas, yet, by its nature is hindered from attacking at one time the entire skin, as an interval must elapse before a second ring can follow the first. In point of fact, in *tinea circinata*, though there may be several rings in existence at one time, and some of them include a very large area, yet we seldom have to deal with surfaces more than six inches in diameter, usually with much smaller.

The disease advances over the skin at about the rate of a quarter of an inch weekly; this is about the rate of progress in *tinea circinata* also. As advancing rings spread, their regularity is modified by the shape of the parts, the nature of the skin they travel over, and by encountering other systems of rings. Thus, after a time, the plan is lost or obscured, while the pattern of the disease, so to speak, is everywhere preserved.

In fair-skinned races, chloasma, or pityriasis versi-color, shows as a brown or fawn-coloured patch on a light ground. In the dark-skinned races, on the contrary, it shows as a lighter coloured patch on a dark ground. In the yellow-skinned races, like the Chinese, in some the colour of the patch of disease and general complexion so nearly correspond that it is only by observing the scaliness and slight elevation of the part, and by the use of the microscope, that we can pronounce it chloasma. In coolies, and those whose skin is darkened by exposure to the weather, the spot is always much paler than the healthy skin; in the pale, sallow-faced shop-keeper, always darker than the healthy skin. A very large proportion of the natives of this district can show patches of chloasma, usually about the neck, chest, or shoulders, or over the abdomen just under the waist-belt. Every

one is familiar with the mottled appearance the skin of
coolies frequently presents. I have satisfied myself
that this is chloasma, and is entirely owing to the
microsporon furfur, which can be found in great abundance in any of these cases. The fungus I have
contrasted with that from cases of chloasma brought
from Europe and America, and find them to be
identical. It is situated on the under surface of the
outermost pellicle of epidermis, and the spherical,
double-outlined conidia, arranged in clusters, and
short much-jointed mycelium are quite characteristic.
The colour of the chloasma spot is owing to the colour
of the fungus, and not of the skin; and being the
same or nearly the same in every case, it appears
lighter than the skin in dark races, and darker than
the skin in fair races.

Limited Geographical Area within which Tinea Imbricata
Flourishes.

An additional argument for separating this disease
from *tinea circinata* and placing it as a species by
itself, is supplied by the peculiarity of its geographical
distribution. I have seen a great many cases in Amoy,
but, with one exception, all of these have been at
one time in the Straits of Malacca, or islands of the
Malay Archipelago, and it was there the disease was
acquired. I have seen cases in South Formosa also,
but as I made no inquiries as to where their skin-
affection was acquired, I cannot say whether it was
indigenous or imported. For a considerable part of
the year the climate of South Formosa is very like
that of the Straits. The instance I refer to as having
arisen in Amoy was in the person of the relative of

a man who had returned from the Straits covered with the disease. Disregarding this case, it would appear that some peculiarity of climate is necessary for the ready spread of the disease from person to person, although when once established in the individual it flourishes in China as well as in its home, as proven by the results of inoculation. Possibly, in the warm, moist, equable climate of the Straits, there is developed some fungus element which will not grow in the colder, drier climate of China, and the spontaneous spread of the disease is effected by this.

I believe that *tinea imbricata* is the disease described as " Pita," or " Tokelau itch," in the " Scheme for obtaining a Better Knowledge of the Endemic Skin Diseases of India," edited by Drs. Fox and Farquhar, and also alluded to by Dr. Thin in a late "Practitioner." If it is identical with the Samoan disease, we know that it spreads rapidly enough under suitable circumstances. As far as I am aware, there is no other epiphytic skin disease, with the doubtful exception of the fungus foot of India, with so limited a geographical distribution.

Tinea Imbricata the Connecting Link between Chloasma and Tinea Circinata.

Assuming that I have proved the existence of a parasitic skin disease affecting the rete Malpighii, we have now, apart from those confined, or nearly so, to the hairy scalp, three well-marked epiphytic skin diseases, viz. :—*tinea circinata, tinea imbricata,* and *chloasma,* each affecting a different layer or element of the skin. *Tinea circinata* has its seat in or on the corium, or deep layer; *tinea imbricata* in the rete Malpighii, or middle layer; and *chloasma* in the epidermis or surface; and to this selection of locality, rather than to any peculiarity in the habits of their respective fungi, seems to be due the characteristic clinical features of these different diseases. The epidermis, so abundantly and constantly reproduced, supplies a never-failing supply of pabulum for its fungus; so that, while spreading at the margin of the patch, there is no death of fungus or subsidence of the disease in the centre of the part affected, the disease relinquishing no place once attacked. Hence its appearance in a circular patch, uniform in colour and texture throughout its extent. In *tinea circinata*, on the contrary, the fungus, living on some element of the more slowly reproduced corium, while spreading towards hitherto unexhausted, unaffected tissue, is compelled to relinquish what it has already passed over, dying for want of the suitable element; hence it assumes the form of a single ring. *Tinea imbricata* is the link, both in position and appearance, between these two, as the rete Malpighii occupies a place intermediate in position and facility of production between corium and epidermis. The pigment layer is not so easily or rapidly formed as is the epidermis; hence the fungus cannot be universally distributed as a patch over the affected part; but the tissue being more easily and quickly reformed than the corium, the fungus element has the opportunity of starting afresh before from lapse of time or want of food it has completely died out; thus its successive generations advance in succeeding rings.

I am aware that many dermatologists favour the

view that the various skin fungi are but modifications of either penicillum or aspergillus, and of each other, and that the same fungus will give rise to favus, chloasma, or *tinea circinata* according to circumstances. I cannot agree with this opinion.   If it is correct, how comes it that in the same man I can by inoculation, as often as I wish, produce on one arm *tinea circinata* from a case of *tinea circinata*, and at the same time, on the other arm, *tinea imbricata* by inoculating from *tinea imbricata ;* but never *tinea circinata* from *tinea imbricata*, or *vice versâ ?* The diseases, at any rate, whatever may be the nature of their exciting fungi, possess the most essential quality of distinct species— they breed true.

INDEX.

H. K. LEWIS, PRINTER, 136, GOWER STREET, LONDON, W.C.

H. K. LEWIS'S PUBLICATIONS.

A HANDBOOK OF THE THEORY AND PRACTICE OF MEDICINE. By FREDERICK T. ROBERTS, M.D., B.Sc., F.R.C.P., Examiner in Medicine at the Royal College of Surgeons; Professor of Therapeutics in University College; Physician to University College Hospital, and to the Brompton Consumption Hospital, &c. Fifth Edition, with Illustrations, 1 vol., large 8vo, cloth, 21s.

　　⁎ The whole work has been subjected to the most careful and thorough revision by the Author, many chapters having been entirely rewritten, while important alterations and additions have been made throughout. Several new Illustrations have also been introduced.

PRACTICAL HISTOLOGY AND PATHOLOGY: Containing all recent methods used in Staining Bacteria, &c. By HENEAGE GIBBES, M.D., Lecturer on Physiology at Westminster Hospital, &c. Second Edition, crown 8vo, 6s.

A PRACTICAL INTRODUCTION TO MEDICAL ELECTRICITY (with a Compendium of Electrical Treatment translated from the French of DR. ONIMUS). By A. DE WATTEVILLE, M.A., B.Sc., M.R.C.S., Assistant-Physician to the Hospital for Epilepsy and Paralysis; late Electro-Therapeutical Assistant to University College Hospital. Second Edition, 8vo. *[In the Press.*

A HANDBOOK OF THERAPEUTICS. By SYDNEY RINGER, M.D., Professor of Medicine in University College; Physician to University College Hospital, &c. Tenth Edition, revised, 8vo. *[Nearly ready.*

SYPHILIS AND LOCAL CONTAGIOUS DISORDERS. By BERKELEY HILL, M.D. Lond., F.R.C.S., Professor of Clinical Surgery in University College; Surgeon to University College Hospital, and to the Lock Hospital; and ARTHUR COOPER, L.R.C.P., M.R.C.S., Late House-Surgeon to the Lock Hospital, &c. Second Edition, entirely re-written, royal 8vo, 18s.

By the same Authors.

THE STUDENT'S MANUAL OF VENEREAL DISEASES. Being a concise description of those affections and of their treatment. Third Edition, post 8vo, 2s. 6d.

THE ESSENTIALS OF BANDAGING: For Managing Fractures and Dislocations; for administering Ether and Chloroform; and for using other Surgical Apparatus. By BERKELEY HILL, M.B. Lond., F.R.C.S., Professor of Clinical Surgery in University College; Surgeon to University College Hospital, and to the Lock Hospital. Fifth Edition, with Illustrations, revised and much enlarged, fcp. 8vo, 5s.

ON ELECTRO-DIAGNOSIS IN DISEASES OF THE NERVOUS SYSTEM. By A. HUGHES BENNETT, M.D., M.R.C.P., Physician to the Hospital for Epilepsy and Paralysis, Regent's-park, and Assistant-Physician to the Westminster Hospital. With numerous Engravings, 8vo, 8s. 6d.

WHAT TO DO IN CASES OF POISONING. By WILLIAM MURRELL, M.D., Lecturer on Materia Medica and Therapeutics at the Westminster Hospital; Senior Assistant-Physician to the Royal Hospital for Diseases of the Chest. Third Edition, revised and enlarged, 64mo, 2s. 6d.

ELEMENTS OF PRACTICAL MEDICINE. By ALFRED H. CARTER, M.D., Physician to the Queen's Hospital, Birmingham, &c. Second Edition, crown 8vo. *[In the Press.*

LONDON: H. K. LEWIS, 136, GOWER STREET, W.C.

H. K. LEWIS'S PUBLICATIONS.

GERMAN-ENGLISH DICTIONARY OF WORDS AND TERMS USED IN MEDICINE AND ITS COGNATE SCIENCES. By FANCOURT BARNES, M.D., M.R.C.P., Physician to the Chelsea Hospital for Women; Assistant Obstetric Physician to the Great Northern Hospital, &c. Square 12mo, Roxburgh binding, 9s.

CATARRH AND DISEASES OF THE NOSE CAUSING DEAF-NESS. By EDWARD WOAKES, M.D. Lond., Senior Aural Surgeon to the London Hospital, &c. [In the Press.

By the same Author.

ON DEAFNESS, GIDDINESS, AND NOISES IN THE HEAD. Third Edition, with illustrations. [In preparation.

DISEASES OF THE NOSE AND ITS ACCESSORY CAVITIES. By W. SPENCER WATSON, F.R.C.S. Eng., M.B. Lond., Surgeon to the Great Northern Hospital; Surgeon to the Royal South London Ophthalmic Hospital, &c. Profusely illustrated, demy 8vo, 18s.

REFRACTION OF THE EYE: Its Diagnosis, and the Correction of its Errors, with Chapter on Keratoscopy. By A. STANFORD MORTON, M.B., F.R.C.S. Edin., Senior Assistant-Surgeon, Royal South London Ophthalmic Hospital. Second Edition, small 8vo, 2s. 6d.

ON THE BILE, JAUNDICE, AND BILIOUS DISEASES By J. WICKHAM LEGG, F.R.C.P., Assistant-Physician to St. Bartholomew's Hospital, &c. With Illustrations in Chromo-lithography, royal 8vo, 25s.

THE HEART AND ITS DISEASES: with their Treatment, including the Gouty Heart. By J. MILNER FOTHERGILL, M.D., M.R.C.P., Physician to the City of London Hospital for Diseases of the Chest, &c. Second Edition, copiously Illustrated, 8vo, 16s.

NIEMEYER'S TEXT-BOOK OF PRACTICAL MEDICINE. Translated from the Eighth German Edition, by special permission of the Author, by G. H. HUMPHREY, M.D., and C. E. HACKLEY, M.D. Two vols., large 8vo, 36s.

THE SCIENCE AND ART OF MIDWIFERY. By WILLIAM THOMPSON LUSK, A.M., M.D., Professor of Obstetrics and Diseases of Women in the Bellevue Hospital Medical College, &c. With numerous Illustrations, 8vo, 18s.

GENERAL SURGICAL PATHOLOGY AND THERAPEUTICS. By Dr. THEODOR BILLROTH. Translated by C. E. HACKLEY, M.D. New Edition, with 144 Illustrations, 8vo, 18s.

GENERAL PARALYSIS OF THE INSANE. By WILLIAM JULIUS MICKLE, M.D., M.R.C.P. Lond., Member of the Medico-Psychological Association of Great Britain and Ireland; Member of the Clinical Society, London Medical Superintendent, Grove Hall Asylum, London. 8vo, 10s.

PRACTICAL EXERCISES IN PHYSIOLOGY. By J. BURDON-SANDERSON, M.D., LL.D., F.R.S., Jodrell Professor of Physiology in University College, London: with the co-operation of F. J. M. PAGE, B.Sc., W. NORTH, B.A. and A. WALLER, M.D. 8vo, 3s. 6d.

RINGWORM: Its Diagnosis and Treatment. By ALDER SMITH, M.B. Lond., F.R.C.S., Resident Medical Officer, Christ's Hospital, London. Illustrated with Lithographs and Wood Engravings. Second Edition, re-written and enlarged, fcap. 8vo, 4s. 6d.

⁎⁎ *Catalogue of H. K. Lewis's Publications post free on application.*

LONDON: H. K. LEWIS, 136, GOWER STREET, W.C.

.

Ingram Content Group UK Ltd.
Milton Keynes UK
UKHW020838190423
420422UK00006B/425